This
Is
Vital
Information

Also by Dr Karan Rajan

This Book May Save Your Life

This Is Vital Information

DR KARAN RAJAN

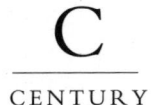

CENTURY

CENTURY

UK | USA | Canada | Ireland | Australia
India | New Zealand | South Africa

Century is part of the Penguin Random House group of companies whose addresses can be found at global.penguinrandomhouse.com

Penguin Random House UK,
One Embassy Gardens, 8 Viaduct Gardens, London SW11 7BW

penguin.co.uk
global.penguinrandomhouse.com

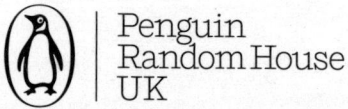

First published 2026
001

Copyright © Dr Karan Rajan 2026
Illustrations © Gwen Burns

The moral right of the author has been asserted

Penguin Random House values and supports copyright. Copyright fuels creativity, encourages diverse voices, promotes freedom of expression and supports a vibrant culture. Thank you for purchasing an authorised edition of this book and for respecting intellectual property laws by not reproducing, scanning or distributing any part of it by any means without permission. You are supporting authors and enabling Penguin Random House to continue to publish books for everyone. No part of this book may be used or reproduced in any manner for the purpose of training artificial intelligence technologies or systems. In accordance with Article 4(3) of the DSM Directive 2019/790, Penguin Random House expressly reserves this work from the text and data mining exception.

Set in 9.75/13.5pt Gill Sans MT Pro
Typeset by Six Red Marbles UK, Thetford, Norfolk

Printed and bound in Great Britain by Clays Ltd, Elcograf S.p.A.

The authorised representative in the EEA is Penguin Random House Ireland,
Morrison Chambers, 32 Nassau Street, Dublin D02 YH68

A CIP catalogue record for this book is available from the British Library

ISBN: 978–1–529–92305–6 (hardback)
ISBN: 978–1–529–13633–3 (trade paperback)

Penguin Random House is committed to a sustainable future for our business, our readers and our planet. This book is made from Forest Stewardship Council® certified paper.

For everyone who ever googled their symptoms at 3 a.m. and wished they hadn't.

For the people who said, 'We don't talk about that.' Sorry. I did.

To every body part that society decided was shameful . . . thanks for still doing your job anyway.

For the patients who told me everything . . . and the ones who told me nothing. You're all in here somewhere.

To the organs and orifices we pretend don't exist . . . this one's for you, too, heroes of the underworld.

And finally for humanity . . . endlessly fascinated by sex, death, and poop, yet somehow still embarrassed by all three.

CONTENTS

1. Go with the gut	1
2. Hygiene matters	35
3. Female health horrors	63
4. Male health hell	95
5. Paging Dr Freud	123
6. Weight loss weirdness	157
7. Body mod mayhem	187
8. Messing with the mind	213
9. The Big C	241
10. Death 2.0	269
Acknowledgements	293
Table of FODMAP foods	295
Index	297

This Is Vital Information

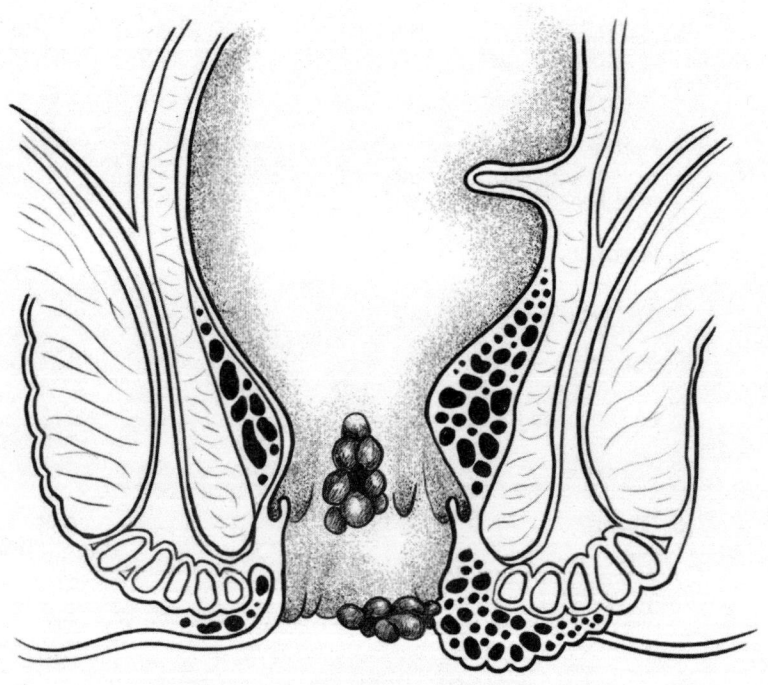

The internal and external haemorrhoids

Chapter 1

GO WITH THE GUT

IT'S 1.30PM. I'm in the hospital canteen feeling stressed and furiously inhaling a bowl of glutinous, nondescript meat. Strictly speaking, I don't even have time for lunch. I'm supposed to be reviewing charts for ten patients. As I wolf down my meal, I try not to think about the number two that's been brewing in the fiery depths of my bowels all day. Now is not the moment to be locked away in the staff toilet attending to my personal requirements.

The meal was meant to be Moroccan lamb stew, but it became perfectly clear that whoever ran the kitchen that day has never actually tasted lamb or anything remotely Moroccan in their life. The regret is immediate, but my body demands calories in any shape or form to fuel me for the next seven hours. The act of ingestion also kick-starts a chain of events within my bowels that slips beyond my control. From here, let me take you through the next few hours:

2.15pm: I feel somewhat full and briefly all seems right in the world. Little do I know I am about to enter a very dark period in my life.

2.45pm: First signs of life. The pressure is growing. An orchestral symphony of borborygmi (fancy doctor speak for gut groans) comes to a crescendo inside me. After consuming lunch, which effectively serves

This Is Vital Information

as drain cleaner, I can feel a loosening within. Even though I'm back on the ward, I have no choice but to make a frantic dash to the toilet. I'm in such a hurry that several nursing staff assume I'm responding to a cardiac arrest alert and fall in behind me. I shake them off with a quick turn of speed and head to the staff toilets.

2.51pm: The internal science experiment inside my flesh pipes has reached boiling point. My gut hates me. I pray there's enough elasticity in my anal sphincters to withstand the barrage of chocolate lava that is about to erupt.

2.53pm: After a seemingly eternal wait, planted on the toilet, we move to a Code Brown situation. At once, a vertical spray of dragon fire is unleashed from my tailpipe. The faecal matter and water mixture that I've given birth to shoots out with such velocity that it ricochets off the back of the toilet bowl and decorates my butt cheeks. I peer down in horror. Is that blood? No, wait. That's last night's pomegranate. Like that makes everything all right.

2.55pm: The sounds are frightening. I'm conducting an auto-exorcism and inadvertently purging my bowels of the demonic entities associated with rancid, unpalatable hospital food. I try to soften the blow by attempting to clench what's left of my arsehole. It proves to be about as effective as holding back a flood with a slice of Swiss cheese.

3.02pm: I hear the door from the corridor open. Footsteps. Then I spot a pair of baby blue nursing shoes outside my toilet cubicle.

'Doctor?' It's one of the nurses I had shaken off earlier. 'Are you OK?'

I dare not reply and just hold my breath as if that activates my cloaking device. The fact is I simply cannot bring myself to be associated with the noxious fumes permeating throughout the restroom. Unfortunately, my attempts to stay silent and invisible are thwarted by the inglorious chorus of unearthly sounds gurgling out of my rear end. That and the shrill noises of my pager as it chooses that moment to kick off.

Go with the gut

'I'm fine,' I lie, despite the fact that I am literally dying from the inside.

The nurse says nothing in response, perhaps momentarily stunned on registering the putrid stench. A moment later, the blue shoes retreat from my view. As the door swings open and shuts once again, I am left cringing to myself and wondering if I'll ever find the courage to leave the cubicle in my lifetime.

While I found the courage to slip out unnoticed shortly afterwards, I did so well aware of the glaring contradictions between my personal toilet habits and my professional life. What had taken place was an atrocity, but only through my eyes and ears. Diarrhoea isn't pleasant for anyone, but it's also just an unfortunate biological process. Moreover, I paid the mortgage by moving other people's guts around, cutting into them, contorting them into different shapes and training them to be better behaved for their owners. From that moment on, I vowed to become more comfortable with my own bowels.

And that is how, dear reader, I came to make it my mission to transform taboo health issues, such as uncontrollable shitting, into watercooler talk.

I faced an uphill task. As you read this sentence, millions of people around the world are evicting brown packages of varying shades from their internal vaults. We're talking about a lot of crap. Despite the plentiful supply of the stuff, we have trouble acknowledging poo. It's almost as if the human race signed a collective NDA to keep bathroom matters private.

As my experience showed, the process of bowel-opening can be associated with the full spectrum of human emotions; from anxiety, despair and embarrassment to panic, relief and even jubilation. Evacuating your bowels pretty much encapsulates what it means to be human, which is why it's so mystifying that this sacred bodily function holds such a diminutive place in our society. Rather than forming the basis of informed discussion and discourse, it is often relegated to childish jokes and downright idiocy. We even refer to it as toilet humour.

This Is Vital Information

Since time immemorial, a major source of disease and death has been transmitted in faecal matter. For most of human history, we defecated in the open while adopting a squat position. As small clusters of humans grew into bustling towns and cities, this quickly became a source of disease and infection. For centuries we did our business in communal cesspits, chamber pots or outdoor privies before toilets were then brought into our homes and their contents conveniently and instantly flushed away. This revolution in toilets didn't just improve sanitation but affected our psychological and social relationship with 'the act'.

Normalising the act of defecation from the exterior to the interior – and notably making it a private affair – turned defecation into an increasingly vulgar act. It became one that provoked disgust, while heralding the onslaught of modern diseases such as haemorrhoids, constipation and pelvic organ prolapse brought on by seated toilets. Conveniently, however, a shit out of sight became a shit out of mind and the basis of so many of our modern-day problems with poo.

Turds may come wrapped in taboos, but they remain a matter of public health and, in some cases, the differences between them can be a question of life and death. Thousands of people a year with all manner of bowel-related disturbances fail to go to the doctor because of their inability to talk openly about poo – a cohort of people are literally dying of embarrassment.

And yet every living human, whether they squat, hover (don't do that), sit or evacuate their innards into a pouch, needs to remove feculent waste from their body. While it might seem like a simple task, the mechanics of human defecation are, in fact, inordinately complex. It is a finely coordinated process requiring the integration of numerous physiological systems including cognitive, hormonal, chemical and neuromuscular signals. It is made up of four phases: basal, when the rectum is empty; pre-expulsive, when stools enter the rectum and the anal muscles keep them there; expulsive, when the anal muscles relax and squeeze the poops out; and end, when the rectum is empty again.

Go with the gut

Defecation is akin to baking a fancy cake. The final product is the culmination of hours of unseen preparation, a biological Willy Wonka factory with internal Oompa-Loompas lurking and slaving away to make the great chocolate biscuit that everyone sees at expulsion.

With such complexity, it's no wonder that defecation-related disorders are commonplace. In fact, a survey conducted by the Rome Foundation involving 73,076 adults from 33 countries and six continents found that 40.3 per cent reported some degree of functional gastrointestinal disorder that influenced their defecation habits.

Although the final production of digestion is expelled from your derrière and is termed 'waste', it isn't necessarily useless. Human excretions are a potent source of health biomarkers; a real-time indicator of general health and inflammation, which can be an indicator of early disease. While many people know the basic 'signs' of a stroke thanks to the public health messaging of 'FAST' (drooping face, weakened arm, slurred speech, time to call 999), the same cannot be said for shit or what it might be telling you.

The fact is almost half of UK adults can't identify what a 'healthy' stool sample looks like and one in four have never checked their poo. At least half of UK adults haven't followed up and actioned their cancer screening invitations and a million do not attend a screening within six months of an invite. Worse still, over a third of adults aren't aware of the warning signs of bowel cancer and one in four admitted they would be too embarrassed to seek medical help for a gut- or poo-related issue. And yet bowel cancer is the second biggest cancer-related killer in the UK and the US.

The scale of this issue truly hit me when I was seeing a patient a number of years ago for 'indigestion'. They described some symptoms – acid reflux, lethargy – and as part of my standard medical history I quizzed them on their bowel habits, not in expectation of anything untoward. I was taken aback when they admitted their stools had been loose for the last six months, with occasional streaks of blood. On examination of their abdomen, I felt a large mass on the right side and immediately organised a CT scan, which revealed an advanced colonic cancer.

As I say to all my patients, if anything doesn't look or feel right or if you've noticed an unexplained change in your bowel habits then you should seek medical advice. When a bowel cancer is caught early, 98 per cent of people will survive a year or more. That drops to under 50 per cent when the cancer is diagnosed at a later, more advanced stage.

We all have a different relationship with our bowel habits but bringing faeces and farts into the open will positively impact our health and welfare.

MAKING FRIENDS WITH FAECES

It's fair to say that the world would be a more relaxed place if we could just accept that shitting is a fact of life. Society has a lot to answer for here, and while it could take a generation for it to become a matter of public discussion, we can make a start here.

Over the course of my career, I have encountered many patients ruined by their bowels and bedevilled by the breakdown of their internal plumbing system. In helping them, I have identified several common factors that can contribute to the malfunction of the waste disposal system and have established some core principles most people can follow to enjoy a healthy, regular and largely successful bowel habit.

Feculent facts

If you're eating or drinking anything at this point you might want to stop. Enjoy that last glug of tea before we get into the nitty gritty of faeces.

Most people wrongly believe that excrement is entirely made up of what you have consumed. But this is not quite true: faeces is mostly water (three-quarters of it, in fact). The water content of faeces is key to ensuring your trouser biscuits are soft enough to slip out with ease. The remaining solid component is a combination of retired gut flora relieved from their digestive duties, indigestible fibres and a slurry of medicinal components, cholesterol and various undigested proteins, fats, a scattering of bile pigments (which contribute to the glorious brown colour), steroids, sloughed-off epithelial cells (the stripped-off biological wallpaper that are the cells lining your intestines), mucus and inorganic minerals.

But the content and consistency of your faeces, as well as its expulsion, are of course all influenced by what you eat and drink. So now we've got the basics covered, let's move on to diet.

The role of diet in dumps

This is not a diet book. I am not a diet zealot. I have not received any funding from Big Vegetable, Big Meat or been influenced by any diet-related bigotry or fanaticism. However, I am a fiend for fibre and prebiotics when it comes to gut health and I shall explain how these help you to form perfect little chocolate parcels that exit your tailpipe but also make your internal environment far more hospitable for your gut microbes.

Prebiotics

You may have heard the term 'prebiotics' thrown around. These are substances that support good gut bacteria and are found in foods like leeks, garlic, onions and asparagus. To be effective, they rely on good bacterial strains already camping inside your gut and if these are present, prebiotic-rich foods help them to flourish and outcompete any 'bad' bacteria that might be present.

When your doctor recommends you eat more fibre, the benefits are more for your bacterial friends than you (although you will ultimately reap the rewards). When the gut microbes are given plenty of dietary fibre to eat, they will churn out vitamins, fatty acids and fine-tune your immune system. The reason why prebiotics are a secret weapon in your arse-nal is because bad bacteria have a hard time processing them and are unable to produce harmful chemicals.

The key to supercharging your dumps is to consume a wide range of prebiotics such as the following (not an exhaustive list):

- **Fructooligosaccharides (FOS):** Short-chain fructose molecules found in foods like onions, garlic, asparagus, bananas

- **Galactooligosaccharides (GOS):** Commonly found in human milk (delivered to babies via breast milk and included in infant formula) and dairy products, this can promote the growth of bifidobacteria

- **Beta-glucan:** A type of prebiotic found in foods like oats or barley. It can help regulate LDL ('bad') cholesterol

- **Resistant starch:** Found in green bananas, cooked and cooled starchy foods like rice, potatoes and pasta – this type of starch isn't digested in the small intestine but facilitates fermentation by lactobacilli in the large intestine.

My favourite go-to source of prebiotics is a herby, garlic potato salad cooked the day before with some boiled pasta and a few pieces of tofu thrown in (which you can substitute with meat or vegetables as desired). These cooked and cooled resistant starches from the pasta and potatoes are gold dust for gut health.

Unfortunately, some of the best prebiotics are also high in FODMAPs (fermentable oligo-, di-, mono-saccharides and polyols), short-chain carbohydrates that can trigger bloating, gas and gut distress in those with IBS (irritable bowel syndrome) or sensitive guts. So, while foods like garlic, asparagus and onions might be gut-nourishing for some, they can be gut-wrecking for others. If high FODMAP prebiotics turn your intestines into a war zone, fear not, there are plenty of gut-friendly, low FODMAP options that still feed beneficial bacteria without the fallout. See page 295 for further information.

Go with the gut

> *Foods to lure the chocolate kraken*
> *(aka the shy poopness monster lurking within)*
>
> Eating foods with high water content like cucumber (96.73 per cent water), iceberg lettuce (95.64 per cent), celery (95.43 per cent) and tomatoes (94.52 per cent) will keep your back garden drainpipe clear of any unwanted debris.
>
> Drink water. Since your lumps of brown gold are about 75–80 per cent H_2O, adequate water intake ensures the stool is soft but well formed and easy to pass – think of a well-baked moist cupcake (sorry).
>
> Have a coffee. People swear by their morning coffee for kick-starting their daily dump – funnily enough we don't know the exact mechanism behind this. The most widely accepted hypothesis is the gastrocolic effect: any food or liquid entering the stomach causes a cascade of digestive secretions and hormones to kick in, including cholecystokinin, which can trigger gut contractions and encourage digestion.

Eating the rainbow for a pot of brown gold

While fibre and water intake is crucial for the health of your gut and bowel function, we now have evidence that the greatest predictor of a healthy gut microbiome is the diversity of plants in one's diet; specifically the consumption of thirty different plants per week.

I know thirty plants a week sounds like a lot, so here's a cheat code.

The good news is that you don't need Peruvian quail eggs, Sumatran sea moss, or ancient Amazonian root extract blessed by your local Instagram wellness influencer. You can do this with normal plants – vegetables, grains, pulses, nuts and fruits – with no second mortgage required. A good variety of these will provide you with polyphenols, like lignans and flavanols, which protect the body's cells from damage, omega-3 fatty acids, which reduce inflammation and help heart and brain function, and the super-healthy fibre beta-glucan.

Here, for example, is my lazy-but-genius high-fibre, plant-rich smoothie. This one smoothie hits at least eight to ten plants in a single go because efficiency is everything when you're trying to hit that thirty-plant diversity flex.

1 banana (resistant starch if slightly green, more sugar if ripe – your call)

1 handful spinach or kale (prebiotic fibre + polyphenols)

½ cup frozen mixed berries (polyphenols + fibre)

1 tbsp flax seeds (omega-3s, lignans, gut-friendly fibre)

1 tbsp chia seeds (soluble + insoluble fibre, gut-boosting magic)

½ cup oats (beta-glucan for heart health + gut fuel)

½ cup unsweetened yoghurt or kefir (probiotics for microbiome diversity)

½ tsp cinnamon (boosts microbiota diversity, fights inflammation)

1 cup almond or oat milk (extra plant points)

½ carrot (grated or chopped; because gut bacteria love variety)

Optional: ½ tsp cocoa powder (because why not sneak in some flavanols and antioxidants?)

Instructions (so easy you can do it half-asleep)

1. Throw everything in a blender

2. Blend until smooth

3. Drink it and feel smug about your fibre intake.

> ### *Other easy wins for gut health and plant diversity*
>
> Spices = phytochemical goldmine. Cinnamon, turmeric, ginger, cumin, mixed herbs all count towards plant diversity. Just throw them into whatever you're cooking.
>
> Seeds and nuts = zero effort, big gains. Sprinkle flax, chia, sunflower, pumpkin, almonds, walnuts on to oats, yoghurt, salads or even toast. They all count as separate plants.
>
> Frozen mixed vegetables = a criminally underrated life hack. Buy a bag of frozen mixed veg and stir it into anything. That's five to six plant foods in one go.
>
> Soup and curry = sneaky plant bombs. Throw in lentils, chickpeas, carrots, spinach, tomatoes, garlic and spices to tick off ten-plus plants in one meal without even trying.

Dropping the kids off at the pool

A bowel motion, a number two, pooing, pooping (if you're American), laying pipe, squeezing out a chocolate log, laying a brick – the act of defecating goes by many names and euphemisms. As a medic, I hear patients tripping over their own tongues in a bid to disguise the fact that they're talking about shitting. As soon as they pause before offering up a substitute, I know exactly what's on their mind. Granted, it's fine if it helps them to tell me the problem. I just wish that we lived in a world that didn't make it compulsory to bring even a shred of self-consciousness or shame to the conversation.

Anxieties about excrement range from the mild to the extreme. Much of this comes down to the sound of the act taking place. Beginner-level embarrassment starts with 'The Flush Hush': using the sound of running water or continuously flushing the toilet to mask the noise of their plops. The art of drowning out groans, moans, toots and tinkles is taken most seriously in Japan. There, to reduce water wastage due to excessive and continuous flushing by embarrassed women wishing to conceal their bodily noises mid-dump, the Japanese toilet maker TOTO invented the Sound Princess: a small device that creates a noise similar to the toilet being flushed. Some of the latest models even have timers and adjustable volumes.

Intermediate-level concealing tactics are best illustrated by the 'poo cushion'. This involves wrapping several layers of toilet roll around the hand to turn it into a paper glove. When deployed with care, it allows the practitioner to catch the faeces before it drops noisily into the water. It's a technique that might spare blushes but comes with a significant risk of solving one problem but creating another.

An 'advanced' technique to conceal your bowel habits includes removing the evidence from the crime scene. This is an act fraught with danger, as highlighted by the 2017 BBC News headline 'Woman trapped in window trying to retrieve poo after Tinder date'. In short, having excused herself to use the bathroom at her date's house, the poor individual at the heart of the story produced a mighty specimen that resisted all attempts to be flushed away. In the harrowing series of events that followed, she resorted to plucking out the poo with careful use of a loo roll with a view to disposing of it out of the window. Unbeknown to her, and to her eternal shame, the window only opened into an air gap formed by another pane of glass. Not only did her efforts to dispatch the evidence see it wedge neatly at the bottom of the gap, but her bid to climb in and remove it also left her trapped like the turd itself. It's a cautionary tale that ends with a call to the emergency services, and an end to a romance before it had reached its first flush.

The final frontier

Occasionally, the stigma associated with poo and the incumbent shame of this natural biological process becomes so overwhelming that it can transcend into a medical condition: parcopresis – doctor speak for shy bowel syndrome.

Go with the gut

Often, I've seen patients who have not opened their bowels for two or three days. In some cases, they've gone for a week without a trip to the toilet. In rare instances, that has extended to a fortnight. One time, I was acquainted with a patient suffering from notably non-compliant bowels. Having shown up in A&E with exquisite abdominal pain and vomiting, they informed me that thirty-two days had passed without a poo. I requested a CT scan, which is a little bit like viewing the patient with superpower vision. What it revealed was a chronically stretched and dilated intestine, filled to the brim with month-old faeces. In the midst of an uncomfortable rectal examination for us both, I felt the human equivalent of cement at the tip of my finger, devoid of all moisture. Diagnosing faecal impaction, and with a long shift ahead of me, I determined that the most straightforward solution was a manual evacuation.

With the patient under a general anaesthetic, and their legs splayed up in the air to give the best possible exposure of the orifice of doom, I found myself going to work equipped with a sterile metal spoon. After thirty minutes of unenviable scooping, breaking down and excavating, I unearthed not precious treasure but a month's worth of stools. On coming round, the patient was as relieved as I was to have put the ordeal behind them. Even so, they were less than forthcoming about how they had arrived in this condition in the first place. All I could determine was they lived in a place with a communal toilet. The fear of pooping, or more importantly the perceived *embarrassment* that it would cause them, prevented regular visits to the toilet. As a result, a kind of defecation denial had evolved, which resulted in me being unable to face dessert for some time afterwards.

How to banish the bathroom blues

So it's that time again. Your rectum is stretched beyond comfort signalling for you to empty your heavy cargo into the nearest flushable receptacle. You're comfortable doing the business on your own throne but when it comes to sharing your biological waste with the rest of the world, public toilets are a challenge too great. It mires you in anxiety and has you stalling.

I will admit I've had to overcome my own inhibitions with this in the past. Simply put, public places like schools, hospitals and offices aren't conducive to good digestive or colonic health, with sandpaper-like toilet paper, doors that don't fully cover gaps, poor ventilation, inadequate cleaning, the embarrassment of toilet neighbours . . . the list goes on. While most people have to face these dilemmas at some point – and I doubt anyone of sound mind actually enjoys the fanfare of shitting in public – if you desperately struggle with the above you might well have parcopresis, an inability to poop in public that can drive you potty.

Some sufferers of this unfortunate condition report freezing mid-poo upon hearing someone enter the toilets, requiring utmost shrine-like silence before recommencing their rectal prayers. For some, this fear even extends to peeing (known as paruresis, or shy bladder syndrome).

If left untreated, shy bowel syndrome can wreak untold havoc on one's sanity and bowels and seriously impact their quality of life. Relationships, social lives and job management all suffer as a result. In the worst cases, such lethal shyness can lead to anxiety disorders or even agoraphobia – the fear of leaving your house to avoid such situations.

There may be a range of mental or physical reasons behind this, so discussing the issue with a healthcare provider might result in a solution, ranging from counselling to a more practical workaround. For example, if you know that dairy products do a number on your number twos, you could try avoiding dairy before you go out or you could book a medical consultation to check for a lactose allergy. Keeping a food diary to identify food–bowel associations is key in this situation.

Another strategy could involve a gradual, gentle exposure to public toilets. Perhaps you could use an empty public toilet at night-time when it's empty, then at off-peak hours, until finally you're comfortable relieving any kind of bowel urge during the 8.30 rush.

Your poo routine

A common question posed to me by netizens of the online world — and the real patients I have seen in my surgical clinics — is what constitutes a normal poo routine?

Humans like to conform (most of the time) and it's only natural that people want to know how their pooing patterns compare to others. I suspect most people assume that 'normal' means going once a day. Having seen thousands of patients over the years, I've learned that normal is not an exact number but varies within a range known as the 'Goldilocks zone'. This means if you empty your bowels between three times a day and three times a week, your range is 'just right'.

However, this takes into account only quantitative data, as in the number of plops you perform, and not the equally important qualitative information, namely: how easy is it for you to pass your stool? Are you straining, grunting, sweating and groaning, or is it literally dropping out like slop from a bucket? There are any number of reasons why this might be happening but constipation might be your first port of call.

The ultimate guide to constipation

Constipation is hard work. It combines the frustration of waiting for a train that's facing unexpected delays with a hint of fear that you're now going to be late for work, which usually makes the situation worse. You could attempt to bypass the system and use excessive force to deliver a fresh baby turd into the world but often all you are left with is something resembling rabbit pellets.

Constipation usually occurs when the enteric nervous system (the nerve supply of the gut) and the hardware of the gut (the muscles) don't work together to empty your gut effectively.

Your time spent on the toilet should be glorious solace but for those who hold the constipation club card, it is an agonising journey through the tenth circle of hell. Constipation is less about the frequency and more about the difficulty of passing a motion and can cover an entire spectrum. Most people have likely endured a brief bout of constipation due to periods of travelling, side effects of medication (such as iron tablets), illness or even stress. Longer-term constipation, though, can be the result of pelvic floor issues, gut diseases, neuro-psychological issues, poor diet or chronic poor toilet hygiene practices.

For most people, constipation is a transient issue. While the gut can be an unpredictable and ferocious beast, it is more often than not a creature of habit. The gut brain (the enteric nervous system) knows and remembers your food preferences, your toilet schedule, your water consumption, your activity levels – heck, it even knows the time of day thanks to built-in mini circadian clocks within every cell in the gut.

In case of pooping emergency, read this

I like to break down constipation treatments into two distinct categories.

The first category is 'mush'. These are treatments that work by drawing water into the intestines, making the contents softer, lubricating the lining and helping things move along the digestive tract. In other words, it makes your poop 'mushy' (psyllium, lactulose, sorbitol (as mentioned below), magnesium, etc.).

The second major category is 'push'. These are things that stimulate your gut and push things along your intestines by causing contractions of the colon (senna, Dulcolax, coffee).

Things in the mush category can be used as long-term options and regularly. Push category foods are a 'break glass in case of emergency' option.

Or you could try . . .

Bathroom yoga. You can do this biological human twister or toilet acrobatics while sitting on the throne. By crossing one leg over the other, it mimics the same internal physics of a squat and relaxes your pelvic floor to help you evacuate easier.

Come in, put your feet up. Foot stools are a game-changer for pretty much anyone. If you don't want to buy one of these, you can simply roll up an old towel and put it under your feet when sitting on the loo. Whichever way you do it, elevating your feet so your knees are slightly higher than your hips helps to straighten your rectum and reduce straining.

Emergency fruit salad. If you're in need of something to ensure a smooth ride on the Hershey Highway look to natural 'laxatives' found in some common foods. Pears, prunes and plums contain a substance called sorbitol. This is a sugar alcohol that acts as a natural laxative by drawing water into the colon, softening the stool and making it easier to pass.

Also consider adding kiwis to the mix if you're hoping to get things moving. Kiwis contain an enzyme called actinidin which increases gut motility – essentially speeding up the colonic transit. It also helps to break down proteins to make digestion easier. And if you eat kiwis with the skin on, you get 50 per cent more fibre.

The poo normal

We've touched on how often, but what else is 'normal' when it comes to pooing? In general terms, a satisfactory toilet motion should be brief, effortless, complete and somewhat prompt. How often you go is not as important as how easily you go and how completely you go. Just don't lose sight of the fact that our flesh pipes and internal tubings are all wired differently. You may go more than three times a day with perfectly formed stools unaccompanied by any symptoms – largely due to a high fibre diet – and equally you may only go twice a week but with easy to pass large bowel motions. Technically these numbers would be considered outliers but that doesn't mean something is 'wrong'.

Generally, defecation only becomes a problem if it feels like a problem for you.

Other factors, such as the odour of your chocolate deposits, might concern you. If something smells that horrific, for example, then it must be an external manifestation of internal anarchy? Again, not necessarily. Some conditions, such as certain food intolerances, are associated with volatile aromas, but typically patients complain of other symptoms before the smell of their output. On the whole, the smell of the average person's waste – no matter how putrid or toxic – bears little relation to overall gut health.

The rectum: a glass half filled

The rectum, where faeces is stored before expulsion, is an incredible biosensor or, to be more precise, an effective pressure detector, because it is eerily accurate at detecting its own degree of emptiness.

In fact, the recto-anal inhibitory reflex has likely saved you from countless mishaps. When it works, this reflex means that when faeces descends into the lower rectum in anticipation of its imminent evacuation, the internal anal sphincter muscle reflexively relaxes. This allows the rectum to adopt a more open shape for the bowel action to follow. Since we do not have conscious control over the internal anal sphincter, we rely on the recto-anal inhibitory reflex to ensure that the internal sphincter is only relaxed as the stool approaches.

Of course, if we fail to completely empty the rectum and instead leave the bathroom with even a small amount of retained faeces within the lower rectum, the internal anal sphincter remains relaxed in anticipation of the prospect of further rectal emptying. Horrifyingly, this can result in leakage. It's more likely to occur if the retained faeces is soft and we engage in physical exertion. This raises pressure in the abdomen and literally squeezes the faecal residue like toothpaste out of a tube. Such passive faecal soiling can cause irritation, itching and soreness and also be foul smelling. It can leave sufferers with extreme anxiety and fear of going out in public or socialising.

Shit holidays

There's nothing worse than sampling new foods on holiday or on a work trip abroad only to fall victim to the dreaded traveller's diarrhoea, aka Delhi belly or Montezuma's revenge. So, in order to preserve your bowel habits, let me teach you how to prepare your body to feast on the local food without having to learn the French for 'Do you have any Imodium?'

Every foreign location offers up its own unique food choices. With different geography comes environmental diversity, and that includes a new array of gut bugs. The souvenir you bring back from a different place may include microscopic microbiome inhabitants from your exotic destination.

The gut micro-organisms that reside in the depths of your bowels include bacteria, as well as fungi, viruses and a single-celled organism called archaea. The population make-up is determined by geography and diet (and to some degree time zones and stress).

A significant proportion of the gut bacteria is derived from the various foods we consume. Other countries may have different ways of making or sourcing food, along with its own unique bacterial strains. So, when we feast on new local foods, those unique strains enter our innards in an attempt at colonisation. The rapid dietary changes as you gulp down copious amounts of foreign fancies means your existing microbes are subject to numerous different strains attempting to settle in your gut at the same time. The sudden influx of new bacteria will disrupt the status quo of your gut as it recalibrates, which can result in loose stools and digestive disturbances.

In addition, eating poorly prepared food can pose a higher risk of ingesting pathogenic bacterial strains like E. coli or salmonella. If these colonise your gut, they can cause violent diarrhoea.

This Is Vital Information

The good news is that there are ways to steel your stomach and 'prepare' yourself for a potential invasion. From a microbiome perspective, it takes approximately three days for your gut to stabilise. Start by prioritising freshly washed local fruits and vegetables (sources rich in prebiotic fibre) in the first couple of days. This can help to nourish your existing bacteria as well as gently introduce your gut to newer strains and digestible compounds. Also seek out foods high in probiotics (yoghurt and cheese), which can help to expose your gut to local microscopic hosts.

With so many different bacterial strains competing for real estate and nutrients, doing your bit to ensure the good ones win helps you avoid spending your entire trip in the shit pits. Even then, don't go overboard with the abundant new food choices on offer. Go gently to steadily expose your gut bacteria to the various nutrients and digestible compounds.

Common poo problems

When crapping goes wrong, or doesn't seem right, too many of us pretend it isn't happening. The trouble is we're ignoring potential health issues, many of which can be easily treated. Here are the common problems explained, so you don't have to lie awake at night with worry.

Haemorrhoids

If you're reading this, you have them. Despite the negative connotations of the word, everyone lives with haemorrhoids, the blood-filled water balloons in the lower rectum that help to control your bowel motions.

Haemorrhoids are nothing more than a fancy name for cushions of blood that line the top and bottom of the anal canal. They are a normal part of our bodies and the unsung heroes that help to form a natural seal for your backdoor orifice. Protecting the anal sphincter muscle, they assist in keeping the anus closed during bouts of increased abdominal pressure – in other words, they keep your pants dry whenever you need to cough or sneeze.

Go with the gut

We should all learn to love our haemorrhoids because preventing anal leakage is no mean feat! In fact, haemorrhoids are likely involved in the recto-anal inhibitory reflex, which is critical in helping your rectum determine the difference between gas, solid and liquid. These sensitive haemorrhoids play a role in giving your farts the all-clear to exit the exhaust pipes.

When they are working, haemorrhoids are an example of nature's engineering at its finest, until one of the gaskets blows. Excessive pressure in the body as a result of vigorous straining during bowel motions, pregnancy and being overweight can increase the risk of haemorrhoidal disease. This sees the normal-sized anal cushions dilate and grow, which can cause pain, itching and bleeding. When these veins become engorged and the tissues tethering them in place weaken, the haemorrhoids can flop out, getting their moment in the spotlight – but not in a good way.

Doctors previously thought the cause of haemorrhoids was a closed case – blaming a miserable low-fibre diet and constipation – but studies have suggested there is more nuance to this. A high-fibre diet is definitely one of the recommendations that lowers your risk but it isn't a golden bullet. If you're ramping up your fibre but still not seeing an easy passage of your stool or you are straining excessively, perhaps consider speaking to a pelvic floor physiotherapist or a gastroenterologist, because persistent haemorrhoids might point to something beyond diet. Issues like pelvic floor dysfunction, chronic straining, prolonged toilet sitting, or even structural problems in the anal cushions could all be the thorn in your bottom. In some cases, conditions like rectal prolapse, fissures, or inflammatory bowel disease can mimic or worsen haemorrhoids and a specialist can assess whether you need targeted pelvic floor exercises, posture adjustments, biofeedback therapy, or, in severe cases, medical or surgical intervention.

Pun well and truly intended but the bottom line is that fibre helps – but it's not magic. If the plumbing is faulty, no amount of bran flakes will fix your pipes.

Problematic haemorrhoids are generally caused by straining, hard stools and constipation, but not exclusively. Spending too much time on the toilet, perhaps as a result of scrolling through social media, can also increase the risk of haemorrhoid issues.

Before you blame your bum grapes on doom scrolling, a pre-TikTok 1989 study in the *Lancet* showed that people with symptomatic haemorrhoids spent longer on the toilet reading than those without haemorrhoids! Clearly, the human urge to while away time on the toilet is a tale as old as time. So when you're in the toilet doing the business, focus on the real job at hand instead of extending your Duolingo streak.

My top tips for dealing with haemorrhoids at home

- Consider topping up your dietary fibre with supplements like psyllium husk. There's evidence that this can reduce the risk of rectal bleeding caused by haemorrhoids by up to 50 per cent. You can buy it in powder form and it is easy to add to yoghurts and smoothies.

- If your haemorrhoids are painful, consider using wet wipes or a bidet if you have access to one, as they're far gentler on your balloon knot than harsh abrasive toilet paper, which can leave you with a nasty case of polished ass syndrome, unofficially.

- Try a sitz bath, which is a warm, shallow bath in which you can sit and immerse your derrière for up to ten minutes. The warm water can reduce the inflammation in your bottom and provide symptomatic relief. You can do this multiple times a day.

If your haemorrhoids don't disappear with these at-home measures, you can speak to a doctor about surgery. Interestingly, like many aspects of medicine, our treatment of haemorrhoids hasn't changed much in about 2,000 years. The Greek physician Hippocrates treated haemorrhoids in the fourth century by using ligation to cut off the blood supply; rubber band ligation is something frequently done in outpatient clinics to this day. Though the mere thought of this may send a shiver down your spine, the procedure is safe, simple and pain free. And the benefits far outweigh the slight awkwardness of speaking to your GP.

Irritable bowel syndrome

Frequent, crampy bowel motions? Abdominal pain relieved by defecation? Intermittent episodes of no bowel action sandwiched between marathon toilet sessions where you seem to spend all day on the throne? An urgent need to defecate after eating, particularly after meals high in fibre or fat? Welcome to the world of irritable bowel syndrome (IBS).

There exists a large, hidden cohort of people out there who may well have IBS and simply put up with their unruly intestines. At the heart of IBS is a disorder of the gut–brain interaction. It's a functional condition because while the bowel may not be acting politely, there is no visible, structural or objectively measurable cause.

IBS is fairly common, with around 10 per cent of the global population affected by their rebellious, unpredictable, teenager-like bowels. And unfortunately, just like those hormone-fuelled teens, IBS is something of a mystery because we haven't pinpointed exactly what causes it. Interestingly it is less likely to occur in the over-fifties demographic and affects more women than men.

How long have we known about IBS? The earliest account we have of it dates back to 1892, when the moustachioed, spectacle-wearing Canadian physician William Osler described a strange condition called 'mucous colitis', which encompassed a mixture of abdominal pain and mucus passage via the stool.

IBS is a group of symptoms that can occur concurrently: abdominal pain alongside a change in bowel habit (be it diarrhoea, constipation or a mix of both). The picture of this can change over time, as can the symptoms. IBS is typically a lifelong condition with no single known cure, but luckily it can be managed to the point of ensuring it has minimal to no impact on your quality of life.

As the saying goes for many conditions, no two diagnoses are ever the same. If you've met one person with IBS, you've met one type of IBS; one person may experience abdominal pain as sharp intermittent pains, others may experience wave-like contractions or even burning.

While we cannot use imaging, blood tests or faecal analysis to confirm or exclude IBS, there are patterns of symptoms that fit criteria – in the case of IBS, these are the Rome criteria (named after the Rome Foundation).

To qualify for this club your diagnosis needs to include a recurrent abdominal pain (once a week in the last three months minimum), along with at least two changes relating to bowel habits (such as an improvement of symptoms after opening your bowels or a change in stool form or appearance).

The symptoms of IBS mimic a whole range of other, more serious conditions, which is why doctors will screen you for red-flag symptoms like weight loss, anaemia, and blood in the stool to exclude other diagnoses such as cancer or IBD (inflammatory bowel disease).

All in your head?

For a long time, the medical community was convinced that IBS was a 'supratentorial' condition, meaning it was all in the mind and predominantly caused by stress and anxiety. This led to the misconception that IBS wasn't a 'real' condition – essentially gaslighting patients into thinking they were causing their own symptoms through stress and anxiety.

The thinking now is that physiological changes – so changes to the body – underpin IBS, but the above is not *totally* wrong. There is a neurological aspect to IBS and stress can manifest physically in the gut and contribute to abnormal bodily functions.

So is stress the cause or effect of an 'unhappy' gut?

Data suggests stress can exacerbate and trigger symptoms, which can improve when the source of stress is eliminated. However, studies also suggest that IBS patients are more likely to have depression, higher levels of anxiety and certain phobias – it's a chicken and egg situation. A 2021 study of more than 50,000 IBS sufferers globally found that IBS-ers were more likely to have anxiety.

Treating IBS

A note of caution here: treatment for IBS should be tailored to each individual. If no two cases are the same, then neither are their treatments. There are, however, some generic rules most IBS sufferers may find beneficial, such as cutting out alcohol, fatty foods, caffeine and very spicy food items.

There is also the low FODMAP diet.

Essentially there are different types of sugars that are hard to absorb in the small intestine. A low FODMAP diet involves cutting back or temporarily eliminating these foods. Keeping a food diary can help identify which foods might be linked to worsening symptoms as this can differ from person to person.

The nerve of it all

You're probably quite proud of the deeply wrinkled hunk of electrified fat we call the brain. It manifests thoughts of philosophy, art, complex mathematics, moral quandaries, and is even partial to enjoying the odd raccoon meme on social media. Occasionally, though, this supercomputer in your skull malfunctions and is responsible for untold misery.

For much of human history, from its lofty position above your shoulders, the brain has claimed the throne as the ruler of the human body. However, over the last decade or so novel research is forcing us to consider a new contender from the most unlikely of places: a place that produces curious smells, awkward sounds and steaming hot brown parcels – your gut.

The gut, we now know, possesses a vast and complex nervous system known as the 'gut brain', which can function autonomously and independently of the brain.

These two brains, one in your head and the other in your belly, are connected like two distant pen pals and have a two-way communication stream via the vagus nerve so that the gut can influence the brain and vice versa. This large nerve travels from the brain through the diaphragm and straight into the digestive system like a biological telephone wire, allowing constant communication between your body's CEO and the company employees at a distant branch.

The CEO is shielded from the outside world by the skull, insulated by layers of thick membranes, and safeguarded by a blood-filtering system (the blood brain barrier), effectively isolated from the happenings inside the body.

The gut, on the other hand, is at the coal face, where food meets intestinal lining, where molecules from the external environment are probed by inquisitive gut receptors, and where the gut immune system patrols for foreign invaders and delinquents. This cacophony of information gathered by the gut via its nervous system is fed back to the brain to paint a picture of internal goings on to allow the brain to generate a response.

Naturally, the response of the brain is dictated by the quality of the information it receives from the gut and vice versa. This might manifest as a subtle negative effect on the mood when the gut isn't functioning optimally, perhaps during a bout of constipation. Or going the other way, a period of stress might wreak mild havoc on your toilet routine or appetite.

IBS is one of several intestinal conditions that can occur when the gut–brain connection is disrupted. Interestingly, many practices that benefit the mind can also help IBS sufferers. For example, hypnotherapy or psychotherapy can serve as a form of 'physiotherapy' for your neural network, alleviating abdominal pain in the process.

Sometimes patients with intestinal disorders such as IBS are prescribed antidepressants and patients can be left wondering why. Medications like amitriptyline, for example, affect the brain in the gut not just the one in your cranium, and reduce the symptoms of IBS by influencing the nerves in the enteric nervous system. This makes sense when you consider that up to 90 per cent of serotonin is produced in the gut.

Another well-trodden path to help with IBS symptoms is to make friends with the conductor of the digestive orchestra – the vagus nerve. There is abundant evidence that stimulating the vagus nerve by means of diaphragmatic or deep breathing exercises, with an emphasis on exhalation, can help to induce a state of relaxation in the body and reduce symptoms of IBS.

While an unhappy gut can be a contributing factor (not the sole reason) to an unhappy mind, it's worth noting that we are still figuring out which is the cause and which is the effect. We should not seek to blame depression purely on the brain, gut or extenuating life circumstances; rather we should view it as a wide-ranging condition and consider all factors at play.

As a gut lover, I can confidently say it has a powerful role in modulating our everyday lives, from digestion to mental health and beyond. Sometimes when you're feeling unstuck, just consider whether it's your gut or your brain that needs a session on the doctor's couch.

Dr Google

You might think as a medical professional I would discourage patients from looking things up on Google. In fact, if you're looking at the correct sources and seeking to educate yourself (and not medicating yourself) I encourage it.

However, there is an overwhelming amount of information online that can be contradictory. The issue is that many conditions share similar symptoms so we run the risk of misdiagnosing ourselves, and in some circumstances delaying treatment of a serious illness. If you're ever unsure, the best advice is and will always be to log off and go and see your doctor.

Regardless of what you learn or read about gut health, the digestive system, constipation and related topics, there are certain red-flag signs and symptoms that should prompt you to seek a doctor's opinion. These are: abdominal pain, rectal bleeding, diarrhoea and iron deficiency anaemia.

Do not panic if you've got any of these because on their own the symptoms can cover several benign conditions. The key is in the nuance. If you experience any new symptoms that aren't normal for you, or you experience a sudden change in symptoms or a combination of the above symptoms, then you should get checked out.

FLATULENCE MATTERS

We're talking about farting, the gas from the body's exhaust pipe created in the digestive process. We all do it, but when it comes to blowing off, it can feel as if much of the world around is an Ultra Low Emission Zone. It's another natural act that likes to go by many disguises: dropping a thunder dumpling, eau de colon, anal acoustics, bottom burping, floating an air biscuit . . . No matter how you express it, for the most part farting is considered odious, impolite, uncouth and distasteful.

While farting is generally frowned upon in public, the resulting taboo means we tend not to register what it can tell us about our bodies. Speaking as a surgeon and not a psychopath, I'm not here to encourage you to fart in a crowded room or a lift. At the same time, in an appropriate time and place, you owe it to your health to at least register the notes you've produced to be sure that everything is functioning normally on the inside.

A brief history of passing wind

Despite the negative associations, however, farting has been at the centre of the crudest forms of mirth for centuries. Take the world's oldest recorded joke, which can supposedly be traced back to Sumer in 1900 BC, or southern Iraq in today's money. Stop me if you've heard this one, but it goes: 'Something which has never occurred since time immemorial; a young woman did not fart in her husband's lap'. Laugh? I nearly let rip. The gag might not raise a smile today, but it still tells us that flatulence has played a role in comedy throughout history.

Perhaps the fog of history has blurred our judgement and perception of farting, but it seems like disturbing the air molecules in the vicinity of one's derrière was much less taboo in the annals of history than it is today. So much so that some even made their fortunes from farts.

Take Roland le Sarcere, also known as Roland the Farter; court minster to King Henry II in twelfth-century England. As his name implies, he had one job in the royal court. Every year at Christmas during the festive pageant he performed a bizarre dance that culminated in him farting. For this riotous act, Roland was gifted 100 acres of land and an estate in Suffolk.

We all do it

While your grandmother may deny it, the inescapable biological fact is that everyone farts – we are all slaves to our intestinal gases and anal sphincters. It is simply the result of bacterial fermentation of food, combined with swallowed air and other bodily processes resulting in the accumulation of gases in the intestine. The resultant wind makes its way out through the rectum, vibrating the anal sphincter as it passes. The pressure, velocity and acceleration at the point of exit determines the distinct sounds produced.

The scent of true love

I've consistently maintained that a primary marker of love in a relationship is when you feel comfortable emitting gaseous substances from your tailpipe and dropping trouser biscuits with ease. And just like we put up with our loved one's annoying habits, being full of gas might be a small price to pay for a host of health benefits beneath the surface. We know the foods that produce the most violent noise excursions and pungent odours are rich in nutrients and high in fibre. For all the drama, they also boost levels of beneficial bacteria in your gut. So passing plenty of gas could be an indication that your gut microbes are busy at work keeping you healthy.

Essentially, eating high-fibre, nutrient-rich food is the only route the microbes have to thrive and receive nutrients. If we didn't shower them with love in the form of fibre then your guts would be an arid wasteland. Once they gobble up the fibre you swill down, they create gas and a plethora of molecules (short-chain fatty acids) that can boost your immune system and gut health to protect the lining of your intestines. Just be aware that the greater the diversity of microbial species, the more gas you expel. It's a self-fulfilling prophecy of hot air, but not something to avoid. Rest assured, your farts are generally a symptom of a thriving and well-nourished internal ecosystem.

The magical fruit

But what actually makes you fart more? In 2011, three clinical trials found that over several weeks, half the participants farted more when they consumed pinto beans or baked beans daily. Yes, they really did a study for this.

Interestingly, the initial increase in flatulence experienced by the bean-munching volunteers returned to normal levels after a few weeks as their colons adjusted to the increased bean consumption – a process known as colonic adaptation.

Go with the gut

Along with fibre, beans contain a type of carbohydrate known as an oligosaccharide; in particular, raffinose. Humans lack the enzyme to break down raffinose, but your gut bacteria can and, as they process this carbohydrate, they produce copious amounts of methane, carbon dioxide and hydrogen. Raffinose, however, is an excellent prebiotic fibre, which promotes the growth of good bacteria. Its fart-generating properties can be found in other foods, such as lentils, Brussels sprouts, cabbage and broccoli.

There is a myth that high-protein consumption leads to increased wind generation. However, gastroenterologists and dieticians the world over will tell you that carbohydrates, such as raffinose, are the more likely culprits. If you consume supplements like whey protein, it is more likely that added ingredients such as lactose, fructose or artificial sweeteners are causing your gas. If protein powder with milk or other dairy products causes your stomach to whimper, perhaps check for an undiagnosed lactose intolerance rather than cancelling your gym membership.

Coeliac disease, irritable bowel syndrome and gastroenteritis can cause excessive flatulence, alongside other symptoms, so if there's a distinct change in your flatulence, you can always get yourself checked out. Generally, however, the noxious fumes you produce after eating food, whether it's carbohydrates or anything else, is nothing to worry about and more a sign of a bustling internal metropolis. So toot on!

Sculpting the smell

Medicine has traditionally treated scatological and flatulence science as an ugly stepchild. Occasionally, however, you get a whiff of something interesting. Take the claim that there may be a way to counter the scourge of your rotten fart smell . . .

In 2016, a team of gastroenterologists at Monash University in Australia conducted a study to work out what separates the benign smelling gaseous odours emanating from your behind from the silent but deadly ones. Who says scientists aren't fun?

This Is Vital Information

The team determined that a fart consists of two components: odourless environmental gases from the air we inhale and swallow, and gases formed as a by-product of bacteria fermentation of digested food. Hydrogen sulphide originates from the latter and is responsible for the quintessential rotten egg note in your horrific bottom burp. Importantly, the level of hydrogen sulphide fluctuates depending on your diet. More immediately, hydrogen sulphide in large quantities can be lethal, which might explain why Homo sapiens have evolved such acute olfactory sensitivity to this odour. A typical unpleasant flatus might contain a concentration of hydrogen sulphide in the ballpark of up to three parts per million. A sewage tank on the other hand could contain a hundred times this concentration and could lead to acute respiratory issues if breathed in.

Back to the study. So, examining the faeces of healthy test subjects, the researchers found that mixing it with cysteine (a sulphur compound found in meat, eggs, dairy and other protein sources) caused more than a sevenfold increase in the hellish egg smell. Conversely, mixing the faeces with slowly absorbed carbohydrate sources caused the hydrogen sulphide production to decline significantly as it passed through the small intestine without being fully digested and fermented in the large intestine. These carb sources included resistant starch found in legumes, bananas, potatoes, cereal and fructus commonly found in artichokes, wheat and asparagus. The degree of hydrogen sulphide reduction was near 75 per cent.

So if you're in dire need of minimising your pungent farting fumes for a social occasion, you might want to consider either easing up on cruciferous vegetables in the lead-up to the event (as these contribute to the sulphur component) or you could try an over-the-counter remedy like simethicone. Taking this occasionally is not harmful as it simply traps the gas bubbles in your intestines, but as with any medication over the counter or otherwise you should always consult with your doctor first.

Just be aware that the science on the subject isn't an exact one. Our intestinal chemistry is variable and unique. In a weird way, however, this could be a fun gauntlet to run. You could even engineer your own emission experiment and treat the food you eat like hazardous chemicals for the home fart factory that is your body. Consider it a means to learn more about your own remarkable if despicable internal chemistry.

Now that we've covered the arse-end of your digestive tract, why don't we take a look at the other end of the seemingly endless inner tube – the mouth. This is where the outside world first meets your body, where bacteria can cause havoc, and where hygiene – or lack of it – takes centre stage.

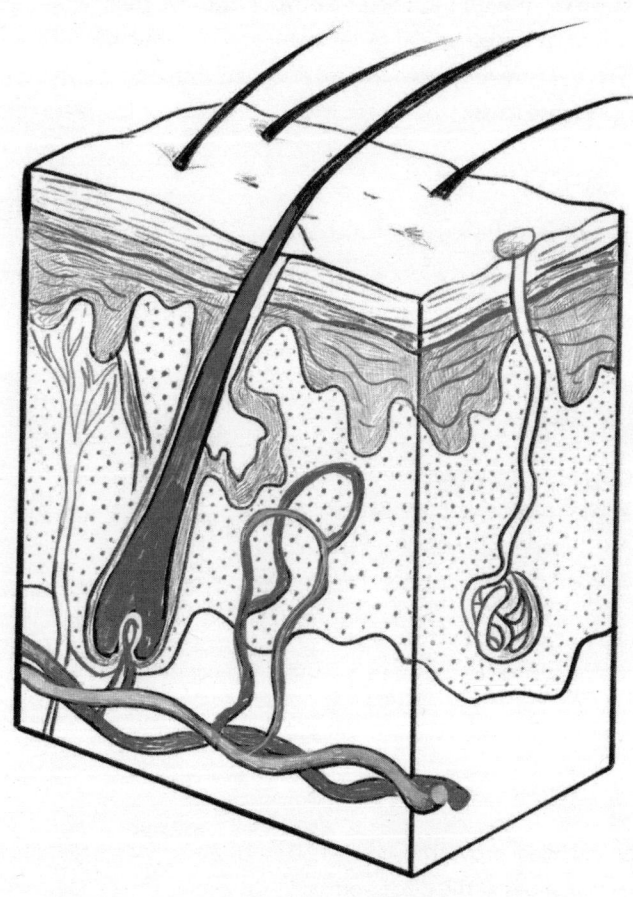

The skin anatomy

Chapter 2

HYGIENE MATTERS

WE FIND OURSELVES IN A WORLD that expects us to scrub up. Indeed, from an early age we're taught how to brush our own teeth, cut our toenails and wash behind our ears. This is all well and good, but as with everything in life we all sit somewhere on a spectrum.

While most of us perform the basics when it comes to personal hygiene, for every soap dodger there is another who can't make it through the day without at least three trips to the shower. Both extremes can create health issues, while those in the middle ground can also find problems strike when they least expect them, not that they would ever admit it.

We might try to cover up issues, from extreme body odour to very bad breath, but in most cases the truth will find a way. Let's look at the worst offenders.

DIRTY TALK

There's an old Hindi proverb that roughly translates to English as 'When you leave your shoes at the door, you leave your worries behind too.'

In the scientific sense, this adage can be translated literally. After all, why would anyone want to potter around the house with a trail of bacteria, grime and dirt from the outside? Growing up in an Indian household, wearing outside shoes inside the house was forbidden. It was treated as a criminal act and if anyone was caught bringing mud or any outside dirt in through the front door, the foundations of the house would practically shake with fury.

The practice of removing shoes at the entrance of a house is not just to maintain cleanliness but has cultural significance. In many Asian and African countries, removing outdoor shoes is a common practice grounded in respect, superstition and hygiene. And science certainly backs up the hygiene argument as studies show that many of the germs brought into households from the environment are faecal bacteria.

Yes, you step in a lot more shit than you realise.

Strength through grottiness

While it's a good idea to keep your surroundings clean, it's important not to go overboard. We now know that not all microbes, or 'dirt', are bad. In fact, some household germs can have a positive effect on children's immune systems as they grow.

A study conducted by the eminent British epidemiologist Professor David Strachan looked at the various factors that influenced the development of immune systems, and the risk of developing allergies. The conclusion was that in households of multiple children, the youngest child often had the lowest rates of allergic disease. The reasoning behind this could well be that the older siblings were bringing home various bacteria and viruses, exposing the youngest sibling to them and bolstering their immune system in the process.

Before you reach the age of three, your immune system is malleable and open to environmental influences. This is why early life exposure to different places and experiences can diversify your microbiome – the vast army of microbes that we all have – which in turn helps to strengthen your immune system. There are landmark studies to support this theory in which it was found that children regularly exposed to dust allergens from animal barns and to livestock have lower rates of allergies. A similar protective effect is seen in early life exposure to dogs and cats – so if you ever need to convince someone to get a furry friend as a pet you have scientific backing.

The great unwashed

One of our first lines of defence against the spread of bacteria is a low-tech offering: handwashing. Now it seems quite normal – and was all the rage during the Covid pandemic – but for a long time, the idea was quite radical, even heretical in the medical field. In fact, it was only in the nineteenth century that the theory that handwashing could reduce the spread of infection in the medical setting first came to light (and it was quickly ignored).

Over the centuries, various faiths have extolled the virtues of handwashing, more for its ritualistic cleansing than for purposes of hygiene, and the practice is mentioned in many ancient religious texts such as the Quran and Talmud.

Of course, those who engaged in ritualistic handwashing would have inadvertently benefited, as was the case during the outbreak of the Black Death throughout much of Europe and Asia in the mid-fourteenth century. European Jews had a lower mortality rate from the contagious bubonic plague than the rest of the population, by as much as half, presumably because Jewish law required their believers to wash their hands several times a day (as well as bury their dead quickly).

But it wasn't until the mid-nineteenth century that handwashing began to be viewed as an effective public health measure within the healthcare field. For this we have to thank the Hungarian physician Ignaz Semmelweis, who in 1846 started an intriguing observational study while working in the obstetric department of Vienna General Hospital.

At the time the leading cause of death among women in childbirth was an infection called puerperal fever, which we now know is caused by the bacterium streptococcus. Before 1823, the mortality rate for mothers during childbirth was around 1 per cent (that is one in 100 women would die when giving birth). That mortality rate climbed from 1% to 7.5% in 1823 after the Vienna hospital stipulated that obstetric doctors and medical students should perform routine autopsies in addition to dealing with obstetric patients. At the same time, Vienna hospital expanded its obstetrics services with a new division that was completely managed by midwives.

Semmelweis, who was working in the non-midwifery obstetric ward, noticed that the mortality rate in his division was substantially higher than in the midwife-only department and decided to investigate.

The mystery behind the sudden increase in maternal death was solved by Semmelweis after one of his colleagues, Jakob Kolletschka, a pathologist, died from an accidental scalpel wound suffered during an autopsy on a woman who had died from puerperal fever. The subsequent autopsy on Kolletschka revealed an infection from puerperal fever. Semmelweis concluded that 'cadaver particles' was the common denominator and were likely to have been on the hands of students and doctors who were dealing with pregnant women. Midwives, on the other hand, were not performing cadaver dissections and were routinely washing their hands, unlike the doctors who rarely washed theirs between autopsies and deliveries.

As a result, Semmelweis initiated a new mandatory handwashing policy in his department using a chloride solution. The rate of puerperal fever and subsequently the maternal death rate rapidly dropped by the year end, from 18.27 per cent to 1.27 per cent.

Despite the overwhelming evidence he presented, Semmelweis's theories were met with scepticism in the medical community. The constant criticism he faced led him to have a breakdown and he was sent to a mental institution. In a cruel twist, he died not long after receiving a cut to his hand – the autopsy revealed his death was caused by blood poisoning. Perhaps if the other doctors had listened to him and washed their hands, this could all have been avoided.

It's easy to dismiss these 'uneducated' medical professionals of the past, but the reality is – as anyone who has spent any time on social media will attest – the war over how often we should be washing ourselves is still going strong today.

The world's dirtiest man

In October 2022, the world learned that a 94-year-old Iranian man had died. He also happened to be 'the world's dirtiest man', having gone without showering or cleaning himself for more than sixty years.

Amou Haji, who lived on the outskirts of Dejgah in southern Iran, believed that cleanliness caused illness and that avoiding bathing was the sole reason he managed to reach his nineties without any health concerns.

Exactly why he avoided water like a vampire avoids garlic is uncertain. Some locals believed he must have had a fear of water due to a traumatic experience earlier in his life. Whatever his reason for this uncleanliness, it mattered very little to Haji who, after all, had made it to the ripe old age of ninety-four despite defying conventional hygiene measures.

Intrigued, a professor of parasitology from the School of Public Health in Tehran conducted a battery of tests on Haji to determine if he had any illnesses that required treatment. He was astonished to find that he had only one detectable illness – trichinosis, a parasitic infection likely acquired from consuming raw or undercooked meat.

The professor concluded that Haji had a well-functioning immune system despite his love of dirt. In an unusual coincidence, after locals finally persuaded him to take a wash in the summer of 2022, he fell ill soon after and passed away.

Perhaps the dirtiest man in the world was on to something here.

Now clearly not everyone would want to, or even should, follow in the footsteps of Haji and interpret this case as a mantra to live your life, but it does beg the question . . .

Do you need to shower every day?

The great question of our times, one that causes fierce debate on social media and can even end relationships. It seems, though, that our need to shower and bathe frequently is based more on a social contract than a mandatory medical requirement.

While some people need a morning shower to wake up and feel refreshed, it may not be strictly necessary. Handwashing certainly limits the spread of germs, but the jury is out on daily showers. In fact, at times it can even be counterproductive as frequent showers can dry out the skin and disrupt your immune system and natural microbiome. Is it time to save your water bill and dial back on your steaming hot morning shower?

Personally, as someone who goes to the gym a few times a week and spends most of their days in close proximity with patients, I shower *at least* once a day, and sometimes more if I happen to be at the receiving end of bodily fluids at work – exploding stomas, a sharp jet of blood from an artery, or some runaway urine deflected from a catheter. You get the idea.

But I am open to exploring more about the idea of 'deshowering' and whether I am betraying the skin's microbiome by the regularity of my washing. But if I shower less, and am vocal about it, will I be subjected to ridicule and abuse?

In the past we didn't used to wash so frequently and even today there are certain activities – such as camping or attending a music festival – during which it is deemed acceptable not to shower. Beyond the cultural taboo, the expense of products like shampoo and soap, and the environmental cost of water use, what does the science actually say about showering?

First, it's a simple fact that bathing can disrupt the skin's microbiome, the fragile ecosystem of microbes that live on and inside the skin. These microbes are your long-lost freeloading relatives, but they are benign as they only feast on what you discard – oils and sweat that build up on your skin surface. Some are beneficial as they stop more harmful infections.

Ultimately, when it comes to showering, we need to untangle hygiene versus cleansing. Hygiene refers to the removal of bodily fluids such as vomit, mucus and faeces, an evidence-backed measure to reduce the risk of transmitting disease. Cleansing, meanwhile, is more ritualistic: combing your hair, wearing deodorant – these don't have any ties to health or reducing disease transmission, although forgoing them might raise your risk of social exclusion.

The fact is, when it comes to how often we should be showering, there isn't a simple answer. There are certain times when perhaps we should seek to shower at least once a day: if you're very active, your job exposes you to agents you need to clean off, or you have certain conditions that cause sweat, oil or bacteria to build up.

There are certain body parts, of course, that benefit from being regularly freshened and cleansed – such as your face, armpits, genital regions and your butt crack to prevent faecal residue collecting there and causing pruritus ani (doctor speak for an itchy bum).

Up your shower game

Wherever you land on the great shower debate, there are some basic principles we should all be following:

- **Short and sweet:** A long shower can feel like the perfect tonic after a hard day at work. As good as it feels, long showers in fact disrupt the skin's natural barriers and increase your risk of irritation. Try to limit your shower time to 3–5 minutes.

- **Some like it hot:** A hot shower might feel therapeutic, while a cold one can be invigorating. The ideal temperature, though, is somewhere in the middle. A mildly warm shower gives you the hygienic benefits of a hot shower, but prevents your skin from drying out.

- **Products:** The soap we use in showers can help to wash away dirt and oil from the skin, right? Shampoo removes oils (sebum) from the hair – also great, surely? Well, when the loss of these natural oils is combined with scalding hot water in your steamy shower this can be the perfect equation for dry skin. When it comes to products, moderation is key.

Moisturise: Moisturising after showering will lock the escaping moisture into your skin.

Eau de BO

Showering does, of course, help to wash away any unsavoury smells – and no one wants to carry the whiff of a rotten egg sandwich. Pungent, foul-smelling odours can trigger nausea, disgust and anger, and give the perception that the offender might be carrying infection or disease.

While this might be the case, a bad case of body odour doesn't necessarily indicate bad health, although the commercial beauty industry might try to convince us otherwise. There is an unlimited choice of products that help us 'get rid' of, or at least mask, our own factory of smells, all of which are quite natural.

In fact, body odour is an essential part of life and we could argue it's even protective. Take the cheesy feet smell; this is driven by the bacteria Bacillus subtilis, which produces antifungal molecules to help keep away other dangerous pathogens. Sweat itself is actually odourless. It is only when other microbes on the skin gorge on some of the chemical compounds in sweat that we get a foul smell.

Sweat helps to cool the body down and body odour carries subtle chemical signals – some people are even attracted or drawn to body odour and it can also signal fear or stress, enabling others to pick up on our emotional state. From a scientific basis, there is no real need to eliminate body odour from our lives, although modern hygiene standards mean most of us are reaching for deodorant or antiperspirant in a bid to keep it at bay. Excessive sweating or a sudden change in body odour might indicate an underlying issue, especially if it's accompanied by other symptoms like weight loss, so see your doctor if you have any concerns.

ORAL 'ORRORS

Of course, nobody would argue that regular brushing of teeth is harmful to health – the mouth can be the entrance to hell without a decent brushing routine. While it's easy to cut corners in our time-pressed lives, the fact is that teeth can quickly bite back. Now, open wide . . .

Tooth be told

You see them frequently. Every time a human parts their lips, you might see one, two or even thirty-two mineral-lacquered nerve fibres dangling in pink flesh adorned by sparkling threads of saliva.

Teeth seem to carry an unfair burden of embarrassment. Unlike most medical issues, which can be neatly hidden under clothes or a poker face, teeth are embarrassingly out there. Every smile, every laugh, every ill-advised yawn during a meeting is a signal to the world: *judge me*. We insist they remain pristine despite years of coffee abuse, midnight chocolate binges and lack of flossing.

Teeth carry a special kind of taboo. We all know we should floss, book the appointments, and maybe not use Diet Coke as a mouthwash – but life gets in the way, and embarrassment builds. The shame snowballs until people are convinced their dentist will judge them more harshly than a court of law. But every neglected tooth tells a story, and the story isn't always laziness. Sometimes it's fear, avoidance, or just the human tendency to hope our problems will quietly go away. Alas, teeth never just go away. They make you pay attention – eventually.

I'm not a doctor of teeth but there's a certain awkward intimacy in being a doctor. You end up examining parts of people they'd rather keep hidden – rashes in unmentionable places, toenails that look like geological formations – and you learn to keep a straight face and your gag reflex under control. But nothing quite compares to the moment you accidentally uncover someone's *tooth shame*.

Black hole

It was supposed to be a simple chest exam. A patient in their thirties, complaining of a persistent cough and coughing up blood. I went through the motions – stethoscope to listen to their chest; a few questions about smoking, pets and the standard history – and then asked them to open their mouth so I could check their oral cavity as part of my examination. And that's when I saw them.

The teeth.

They looked like they'd been holding a grudge against toothpaste. One tooth was missing entirely, another was blackened like it had been on the losing end of a bar brawl, and the rest seemed to have declared independence from each other, marching in different directions as well as multiple points of bleeding at the gums. I managed not to recoil, but the patient must have noticed a micro-expression in my face because they quickly muttered: 'Yeah, I know. I need to see someone about them.'

What followed was a rambling explanation that was less about their lungs and more about their dental history. They hadn't seen a dentist in over a decade. They admitted they'd been chewing on one side of their mouth for two years, carefully dodging anything colder than a lukewarm cup of tea in the hope the problem would fix itself.

It didn't, of course. Teeth are stubborn like that.

Hygiene matters

I suggested they book a dental appointment – not so subtly implying that the 'coughing up blood' might be due to the festering situation in their gums, given the CT scan of their chest was normal. The patient nodded earnestly, though I could tell he was lying in that hopeful way patients do when they're planning to ignore your advice.

As he left, I couldn't help but think about the strange paradox of healthcare: people will let a doctor cut them open, prescribe weird pills, or stick things in unimaginable places, but a fifteen-minute dentist appointment? Too far.

The root of it all

There's a lazy misconception that dentistry and medicine are inherently different even though both are concerned with the health of the body. The last time I checked, the mouth and its contents were definitely part of the body and could be filed under medical.

Dentistry hadn't always been the polished profession of dazzling smiles and pearly whites we know today. Prior to the nineteenth century, it was more of a side hustle for barbers looking to maximise their income. After tidying up a gentleman's beard, the barber would graciously offer to drain a festering abscess, yank out a rotting tooth with all the precision of a blacksmith, or even reset a broken bone if desired. Feeling light-headed? No problem, as they might also throw in a quick bloodletting, too. It was truly the golden age of multitasking, where surviving a haircut was just the beginning of your worries.

It was only when medicine became more specialised that dentistry moved from a hairdressing sideline to more of a medical field. Thereafter, we learned more about how certain diseases could start in the mouth before spreading to the rest of the body. We now know, for example, that oral bacteria and the toxins they produce can be a contributing factor to heart and lung disease, as well as a host of other issues.

Better teeth don't just help us from a health perspective; they do so socially and financially too. Studies suggest that it is harder to find a job or even housing if you have teeth missing due to societal judgement of what your dental health implies about your character. Our oral health can literally change the trajectory of our life, so we should all know a little bit more about what's going on behind our pearly whites.

Mouth guests

The outside world first enters your body through your mouth so it shouldn't be a surprise that it can be the source of many problems arising elsewhere in the body, from infection and influenza to cancer, cardiovascular disease and even dementia.

As your digestive tract is essentially one long twisting pipe, oral bacteria can easily hitch a ride on your dinner and into your stomach and intestines. In most instances, your body has safeguards in place to prevent unwelcome bacteria adapting to the hostile environment of your stomach and further afield. Sometimes they do adapt, however, and studies of bowel cancer patients have revealed that fusobacterium, which is typically found in dental plaque, can colonise cancerous cells in the bowel. They revealed that fusobacterium had a predilection for and attraction to cancer cells, targeting and binding to them.

More studies have shown that fusobacterium can colonise and grow on tumours throughout the entire length of the gastrointestinal (GI) tract and that patients whose tumours were more heavily colonised tended to have worse outcomes from chemotherapy, and a shorter life expectancy as a result. This is an area of ongoing research but in the future it could be that antibacterial mouthwashes will help to improve the outcomes of those with or at risk of bowel cancer.

Oral bugs can also hitch a ride in the respiratory tract, which begins in the mouth and comes to a dead end in the lungs. An overgrowth of oral bugs such as streptococcus pneumoniae and haemophilus infuenzae can lead to lung infections, which in the elderly can often be fatal. In fact, there is evidence to suggest that the practice of good oral hygiene and thorough teeth cleaning among elderly care home residents could reduce pneumonia cases by up to 30 per cent.

The types of bacteria involved in periodontitis – an infection below the visible surface of the gum – can travel throughout the bloodstream and cause chronic inflammation in various organs. Unsurprisingly, periodontitis is linked to a number of chronic states including autoimmune disease, diabetes, cardiovascular disease and even certain cancers.

Once the immune system detects the presence of pathogenic (disease-causing) bacteria it will release pro-inflammatory cellular messaging molecules, which will help to attack them. In the short term, symptoms can appear as swelling, redness and occasionally pain but in the long term, chronic sustained inflammation can develop and cause mischief, in the form of disease.

Poor oral health can also raise your risk of neurodegeneration and cognitive decline. One study of 34,000 patients in the US revealed that those who had lost teeth had a 48 per cent higher risk of cognitive impairment and a 28 per cent higher risk of dementia in comparison to similar individuals who had all their teeth.

And it was all yellow

Modern beauty standards continue to favour perfectly aligned white teeth. In itself this isn't an issue, as vanity is merely one symptom of the human condition that has plagued us since time immemorial. Problems arise, though, when aesthetics trump functional dental health.

White teeth don't automatically indicate good health. Conversely, yellowing teeth are not a sure-fire sign that you're falling apart on the inside. The hue of your teeth is dictated in part by genetics and age, while lifestyle habits such as smoking and drinking can have an impact, as can certain medications and foods like coffee, tea and red wine.

The colour of your teeth is largely down to two of its key components. Enamel (the white that you see on the teeth) is a somewhat translucent outer layer that covers a yellower substance inside called dentine. The thickness of your enamel layer therefore can determine the look and colour of your teeth. Those with thicker enamel can appear to have whiter teeth than those with a thinner outer layer that allows more light to refract through on to the dentine. In the main, this is dictated by genes and not your brushing routine.

Your mouth is bugged

There are hundreds of different species of bacteria in your mouth – indeed, the population runs into the billions in total. Some of the bacteria found in your mouth are similar to those found in the gut and these help with digestive processes and regulate bodily functions. There are also some, such as streptococcus mutans, that are simply malevolent in nature and can attack the enamel coating of your teeth with the lactic acid they produce during metabolism.

Thankfully the rogues are kept in check by other microbes that produce antimicrobial proteins to hinder the growth or harmful bacteria and release alkalis that raise the pH level (the balance between acid and alkaline). As a result, the balance is maintained and generally the community of microbes in your facehole is stable and kept on a leash.

Keeping the pH level of your mouth in check is an important part of protecting your teeth. Generally, the pH level in your mouth should be around 7, a neutral level like pure water. A more acidic level of pH 5.5 and below will cause your teeth to demineralise, increasing the risk of cavity formation. Conditions like xerostomia (dry mouth) or reflux disease can also lead to oral acidity and increase the risk of plaque and cavities. Similarly, medical conditions like Sjögren's syndrome can contribute to dry mouth, as can certain medications like some antihistamines and antidepressants that affect the flow of saliva.

A shift in power

Anything you put in your mouth can alter the delicate balance of good and bad bacteria. Diets lower in fibre and excessively high in carbohydrates and sugars – particularly those in ultra-processed foods – can preferentially feed acid-producing bacteria. These can subsequently thrive in a seemingly hostile environment and outgrow the beneficial bacteria. As a result, the oral pH level becomes more acidic.

This shift in power, when the microbiome in your gut or mouth gets out of balance, is called dysbiosis. All hope is not lost, however, as there are a few simple things you can do to help return your microbiome to a more balanced state.

- Ensure you have an adequate intake of fibre-rich foods. Fruit, vegetables and other types of fibre not only provide nutrients for beneficial oral bacteria to thrive, but fibrous foods, such as carrots or apples, can also act as 'natural toothbrushes', scrubbing away food debris, bacteria and plaque welded on to your teeth, while stimulating saliva.

- Cut back on alcohol (sorry). Alcohol is known to disrupt the oral microbiome by altering the pH level of our saliva, leading to teeth demineralisation and possible cavities. Alcohol can also kill some of the helpful bugs we have in our mouths, including cells around the mucosal lining that lines our mouth and help to protect us against pathogenic bacteria and viruses.

- Don't smoke. Smoking tobacco in traditional cigarettes can lead to stained teeth, bad breath, gum disease and an increased risk of cancer in the mouth, throat, tongue and lips.

- And that also goes for vaping. Marketed as a 'safer' alternative to smoking, studies show that vaping alters the balance of bacteria in the mouth, increasing harmful pathogens like Porphyromonas gingivalis, a major cause of gum disease. In fact, the oral cavity of vapers and their altered oral microbiome is more similar to people with periodontitis (serious gum disease) than non-vapers. Forty-three per cent of vapers show signs of gum inflammation and they are 27 per cent more likely to develop cavities compared to non-vapers due to the high sugar content in some vape liquids and the drying effect of vaping aerosols.

- Don't be tempted to chew tobacco instead of smoking or vaping as it can also raise the risk of oral cancer, irritate your gums and cause tooth decay. A good option is to chew sugar-free gum. This will increase saliva production and balance out the pH levels in your mouth.

- If you use an inhaler, it is especially important you maintain good oral hygiene as some inhalers can reduce saliva production leading to dry mouth and a higher risk of tooth decay or gum disease. After using your inhaler you can rinse out your mouth with water and ensure you regularly brush and floss your teeth.

When should I brush my teeth?

Picture the scene: it's 1am, you've just watched seven episodes of the latest Netflix series and you can feel your eyes starting to give up when you realise you haven't brushed your teeth yet. The thought of leaving the warmth of your bed is all too much to bear and you decide you'll just be extra good with your brushing routine tomorrow. Everything will be all right . . . right?

The fact is, just like you, your mouth is a slave to the twenty-four-hour circadian rhythm and there's a reason your dentist insists on brushing at regular intervals. During the day, your mouth produces more saliva, giving it the optimal pH for the remineralisation of your teeth. At night-time, saliva production comes to a halt and any food products you've squirrelled away in the evening provide nourishment for the harmful bacteria living in your mouth. By the time you've woken up, these bacteria will have enjoyed their all-nighter and need to be eliminated.

When not to brush

OK, so you brush twice a day, floss, you even bought the fancy water floss machine your dentist recommended, and then the doctor you follow on

Hygiene matters

Instagram tells you that actually you're doing too much. *Can* you brush too much?

Unfortunately, there are times when you should avoid brushing your teeth, such as straight after your morning coffee; instead wait at least thirty minutes before your brush your teeth. Coffee is naturally acidic, especially when milk and sugar are added to it, and it can wear down your tooth enamel. If you start brushing before your saliva has been able to restore the natural pH in your mouth, you'll be helping the acidic leftovers get into the nooks and crannies between your teeth. You should also try to finish the coffee as soon as possible rather than sipping coffee throughout the day to give your teeth a break from constant acid attack.

Similarly, if you've just been in the unfortunate position of throwing up, it's understandable that you might want to reach for your toothbrush. However, this is one of the *worst* times to brush as you're just rubbing your stomach acid into your teeth. Yum. Instead, have some water and wait for thirty minutes to an hour before rinsing out with mouthwash.

The great mouthwash debate

Depending on who you ask, mouthwash might be the great saviour of your date night or the cause of all your mouth woes. While it can definitely play an important part in oral health, using it at the wrong time can undermine the hard work you're putting into your dental regime.

What's certain is that you should avoid using mouthwash directly after brushing. All the good work you've done in adding fluoride to your mouth microbiome can quickly come undone by rinsing out with a lower fluoride-content mouthwash. If you do need to use the stuff, avoid anything alcohol-based, which can dry out your mouth and ironically lead to bad breath.

GIVE ME SOME SKIN

Just like the mouth, the skin plays a key part in the body's defence against harmful bacteria. It is the body's largest organ and a remarkable one at that, something I didn't quite fully appreciate when I started my medical training . . .

An elderly man lay on a metal gurney with his face covered by a white cloth. Hs skin was cold to the touch and moist with preservation chemicals to prevent rotting. This was my cadaver in the dissection lab.

Following the instructions of my anatomy tutor, I cut into the middle of the abdomen and began pulling the loosened flaps of skin to expose the deeper layers. The skin was limp and not as supple as fresh skin. Grease from the fat slipped across my surgical gloves.

Once I entered the depths of the abdominal cavity, the skin was relinquished to the recesses of my mind and I ignored it. Instead, I focused on the abdominal organs as well as the various muscles, nerves, blood vessels and bones. Everything was encased within the skin, and yet I just treated it as no more than fancy wrapping material that was quickly torn to reach the gifts beneath.

It was only months later, when I started histology (the study of tissues) and examined the skin under the microscope, that I learned the true complexity of this wrapping and its functions. It was, I discovered, far more than just a biological condom for the human body.

Under the skin

The doctor and author Monty Lyman put it best: the skin truly is 'the Swiss army knife of organs'. It's the unsung hero of the human body that quite literally holds us all together. Here are some of the versatile ways skin can keep you alive and kicking:

- Acts as a terrarium for a wide range of life
- Serves as a thermostat and helps to regulate body temperature

- Provides its own supply of lubrication in the form of sebum from its sebaceous glands
- Performs the role of a blanket via hair follicles that are primed to stand on end to keep you warm when you need it
- Transforms into a walking umbrella when exposed to the sun
- Darkens with pigment to protect your DNA from solar damage.

The skin is the most visible organ we host, and yet it's not as well understood as we like to think. In many ways, it's beautifully mysterious. We sometimes adorn it with decorations, creams, paint and ointments. It reveals feelings, betrays emotion – blushing, sweating and goosebumps – and helps with social communication. It is both a wall and a window, providing a physical barrier against the barrage from the outside world but also playing a key part in forming our psychology and social existence. We learn about the world through physical communication, facilitated by the millions of nerve endings the skin provides, while the skin also offers a lens through which others can see us – for better and sometimes worse.

When it comes to skin hygiene, it's important we define what we mean by hygiene as opposed to 'cleansing' or 'skincare'. Hygiene involves removing matter that could potentially spread disease, from washing hands to remove faeces, vomit or blood, or irrigating and cleaning out wounds. Cleansing removes dirt, oil or make-up from the skin surface – and many products out there claim to give you perfect, younger skin – but most have nothing to do with avoiding disease.

Less is more

Self-care is good. If you enjoy an elaborate ten-step skincare routine and find it relaxing and you enjoy the benefits it provides your skin (and your wallet can fund it) then I'm not here to stop you. However, if you want healthy skin just know that a lengthy, expensive routine isn't necessary for good dermatological health.

This Is Vital Information

I won't judge people for wanting to have great looking skin. It's just that skin doesn't need to look perfect – its main job is to keep you alive. It is the external extension of your immune system and skin issues are often a manifestation of issues in the body or outside of it and topical products are often just a means of papering over the cracks.

Using excessive tinctures, balms and facial treatments does nothing more than strip the natural oils from our skin, before we add moisture back with lotions. The quest for perfect skin is largely unobtainable, although the beauty industry, which likes to play upon our insecurities, might tell you otherwise. It makes us believe there is a product available to deal with natural skin features that have somehow been transformed into taboos. Wrinkles? Oh, buy this cream! Dark spots? This ointment is your go-to. Dry skin? Try this gold face mask that costs a day's wage! It's easy to convince yourself that more is better in your quest for 'perfect' skin.

A pharmacy in your skin

Your skin has an oily layer known as sebum. It acts as a natural sealant to trap moisture and prevent dryness of the skin. Its chemical constituents read like an expensive ingredient list that the best products in the world might use: glycerol, squalene, fatty acids and lipids – you contain an unlimited reusable resource.

A group of substances found naturally in the skin known as natural moisturising factors (NMFs) keep your skin soft and hydrated. These contain ingredients such as glycerin, urea and amino acids, which draw water from the environment and keep corneocytes, aka dead skin cells, hydrated. Yes, the same dead skin cells you might be trying to scrub off with an expensive exfoliant are actually helping your skin function and stay moisturised.

Once these corneocytes have stopped being useful, the skin undergoes desquamation – a fancy way of saying natural shedding. This natural exfoliation happens when microbes feast on dead skin cells. The dead cells act like food for the bacteria, helping them produce beneficial substances like ceramides and peptides after digestion. The bacteria also use sebum – the oil that coats your skin – to keep your skin's oil levels balanced.

Protect and survive

The outer surface of skin is a thin, slightly acidic film known as the acid mantle, made up from a mixture of sebum, sweat, water, dead skin cells and amino acids. Its pH is usually around 4.5, a suitable level to neutralise the threat from most microbial invaders, and it does a great job in protecting your skin from bacteria, pollution and moisture.

The protective shield is also pretty good at sorting itself out. Any products you put on your skin should act as an adjunct to its natural function rather than strangle it into a smooth, sterile, shiny chokehold submission.

In fact, you could try to go without *any* products but if it seems too scary to go cold turkey on your well-tuned skincare ritual, fear not because after roughly a month, your skin microbiome will rebalance and your skin's natural functions will auto-regulate.

I had a long discussion with an experienced dermatologist friend before writing this chapter and asked her what the most common problems she was seeing in her clinics. Her answer came down to the fact that we keep breaking the skin barrier. In simple terms, the skin's natural defences are weakened by excessive cleansing, and this can make it patchy, flaky and sensitive. Unsurprisingly, the compromised barrier can also give rise to or exacerbate eczema, rosacea, psoriasis and even acne.

In short, our obsession with skincare products could spell dermatological disaster.

Reinventing the routine

I briefly mentioned the acid mantle – the protective film of sweat, oils and amino acids – and now here's another reason to look after it. Most foamy face washes are alkaline and will disrupt the acid mantle, raise the pH and encourage the growth of propionibacterium, which can play a role in the formation of various types of acne.

A couple of decades ago, the concept of prebiotics, probiotics and the microbiome were fringe topics and the science world version of a hippie movement. The microbiome is now mainstream. With this in mind, and a greater emphasis on taking care of our microbiome, perhaps it's time we give more love to the *skin* microbiome and modulate our behaviours to avoid eradicating these microbes.

Everyone is increasingly obsessed with gut health and eating probiotic-laden yoghurt. At the same time, we use copious amounts of alcoholic hand sanitiser on our skin. We continue to disregard the science of skin health and view it as a static structure to be plastered with goops and serums or laughably ingesting collagen to increase internal collagen production (it doesn't work by the way; please save your money).

Awful acne

Between the ages of thirteen and sixteen, I must have read every blog, article and magazine that gave advice about spots, and bought every 'acne-fighting' exfoliant, cream or scrub going. Sadly none of them seemed to work, and everything I learned about acne turned out to be plain wrong.

I was lucky in that acne didn't affect me too badly. But as a teenager, a single pimple or boil in my awkward facial real estate had the potential to make me feel self-conscious and embarrassed.

The categorisation of acne as abhorrent is linked to the myth that it's the result of poor hygiene or ill health. The fact is that in many cases the polar opposite may be true. People living with acne often over-scrub their face in a desperate bid to be blemish-free, which sadly can also exacerbate the issue.

Acne is not due to poor hygiene and it is certainly not contagious. It is a complex, multifactorial disease. Genetics are partly to blame, as are hormones, which is why it generally erupts around puberty and improves with age. Local factors such as the microbiome and specific types of bacteria (e.g., cutibacterium acnes) can also play a role.

In many ways, our efforts to completely desterilise the skin can sometimes trigger and exacerbate acne. The fact is people with acne would be better served by visiting a dermatologist rather than taking advice from a beauty blogger.

Take retinoid. This medication is one of the most powerful weapons we have in the war against acne; both in pill form or topical face creams (the latter being better for milder forms of acne). As a bonus, retinoid also works as an anti-ageing, anti-wrinkle cream by stimulating collagen production and promoting cell turnover.

Modern life

Most people have had acne at some point in their lives, regardless of ethnicity or race. Unless, that is, you originate from non-industrialised groups of people in the world. Take the Aché hunter-gatherers of Paraguay, or the Kitavan tribes in Papua New Guinea. For these guys, acne is almost nonexistent, presumably because they've lucked out in the genes department. However, when members of the Kitavan tribe relocate to Westernised areas and adopt Western diets and lifestyles, they often develop acne, which implies that perhaps the habits and vices of modern society have a part to play.

What can we learn from this and what can you do to prevent a break-out?

Diet: The science linking diet and acne is tenuous and inconsistent. What we can say is that acne has a clear association with insulin resistance, which can lead to high blood sugar levels. So if a poor diet and consumption of excess calories leads to obesity – which affects a person's insulin sensitivity – it would also increase the risk of acne. P.S., chocolate does not cause acne.

Exercise: It is well established that regular physical activity can reduce stress and inflammation in addition to boosting the flow of blood to the skin. All these factors in combination may contribute to reducing the formation of acne. In short, our modern sedentary lifestyle may hinder our quest for beautiful skin.

Sunlight: Many of us are exposed to less sunlight due to 9–5 job patterns, which keep us indoors most of the day. The fact is we obtain most of our vitamin D from sunlight. A steroid hormone, vitamin D helps to reduce inflammation in the body, aids healing from wounds as well as fighting off acne-causing bacteria, all of which is good news in battling spots.

Stress: The hustle and grind culture of the modern world leads to stress. Stress takes its toll on the skin indirectly by worsening our sleep patterns as well as driving hormonal imbalances and compromising the immune response – a recipe for acne.

Overcleaning: Skincare products can sometimes lead to acne, or worse break-outs, because they can block pores, irritate the skin (particularly exfoliation) and even trap oil or dry out the skin, throwing the delicate balance of your skin microbiome off kilter.

Science-washing

Let me introduce you to science-washing, a marketing ploy used to transform your perception of commercial products and make them sound more scientific than they are. I promise you, you have most definitely been a victim of science-washing. Use them if they make you feel good. If you have a medical skincare issue, you should see a doctor or dermatologist.

Here are some of my favourite quasi-medical terms used on skin-care products.

'Dermatologist tested': This isn't a certification that something has undergone rigorous industry-standard testing for quality and efficacy endorsed by a body of dermatologists. In all likelihood one or two dermatologists have been paid to check the product for safety and it's usually difficult to verify who these dermatologists were unless the company releases specific details.

'Non-comedogenic' (meaning it won't block pores or cause acne): In real life, sensitivity to skincare products varies from person to person so this is not a guarantee that the product won't worsen your acne. Often trial and error is the only way of finding out.

'Hypoallergenic': No product can promise not to cause an allergic reaction or be 100 per cent safe for eczema-prone or sensitive skin. Your allergy risk will be based on the ingredient list and formal allergy testing or by carefully trying it out for yourself (by applying it to a small area first to check for a reaction).

'Clinically proven': Sounds scientific but often isn't. This phrase just means a bunch of people were given the product and the self-reported changes in certain skin characteristics were noted. There is no guarantee this was done as a controlled study or if any scientific methodology or rigour was applied to the process. If it truly is clinically proven, the gold standard would be to see if there was a randomised controlled trial underpinning these claims.

My rules

Here are my own skincare rules, dermatologically tested (ha) by myself:

- Moisturisers are very helpful for dry skin but they don't add moisture on their own, so it's best to apply them on wet skin to seal in the water. Your skin is pretty waterproof so after around three products are put on your face, not much more will be absorbed by your skin. By the time you get to your fourth, fifth or sixth serum or gel, it's all pretty much bells and whistles and unlikely to do much, if anything at all.

- Beware of 'anti-ageing' products. The ones truly based on science that can help with wrinkles, sun damage and premature ageing of the skin are tretinoin (given on prescription) or adapalene.

- You don't always need to exfoliate. The skin is capable of self-exfoliation if you let it take care of itself.

- Sunscreen should be an essential part of your skincare armoury to prevent age-related wrinkling and reduce your risk of skin cancer.

- Vaseline (petroleum jelly) is an underrated tool. It's cheap and is a pretty effective moisturiser if your skin is dry (if you're not put off by how thick and greasy it is).

- Be patient.

The life cycle of a skin cell is around thirty days. This means that in order to see any noticeable changes you need three cycles of patience to see the new skin cells emerge from the innermost layer of your epidermis (basal layer) to the surface. So if you don't wait for three to six months but instead constantly change your routine and products you won't see the benefits and will likely just irritate your skin and waste money too.

This is apt for most people who do not have clinical skin conditions. If you do, the rules may change and you should 100 per cent be guided by a specialist dermatologist in that condition.

Racist soap

Throughout the nineties and early 2000s, whenever I visited India I would see numerous advertising billboards, TV adverts and posters on bus stops featuring beautiful light-skinned men and women placed next to shampoos and soaps. The words 'white', 'fair' and 'light' were often used to promote the lightening effects of toiletries and beauty products. It came as no surprise that South Asian mothers would tell their children not to go out in the sun too much because they'd get 'too dark'. Thankfully, times are changing and these products have rightly come to be perceived as controversial and racist, but still the taboo persists.

The notion that darker skin tones are dirty while fairer tones are associated with cleanliness and purity is nothing new. In the late nineteenth and early twentieth centuries, and especially during colonial times, some soap manufacturers leaned into this cultural ideology, promoting the 'whitening' quality of soap by showing its ability to 'wash off' the colour of black or brown skin.

While skin-lightening products sadly still exist (especially in parts of Asia and Africa) the marketing of mainstream soap has largely shifted towards 'perfect skin' – clean, blemish-free and glowing. Social media pushes this message heavily and today we're only ever a swipe away from skin-fluencers and celebrities flaunting perfected faces and sharing intricate ten-step skin-care routines. Much of this is, of course, directed at women, who must navigate a labyrinth of misinformation and taboos when it comes to their own bodies.

This Is Vital Information

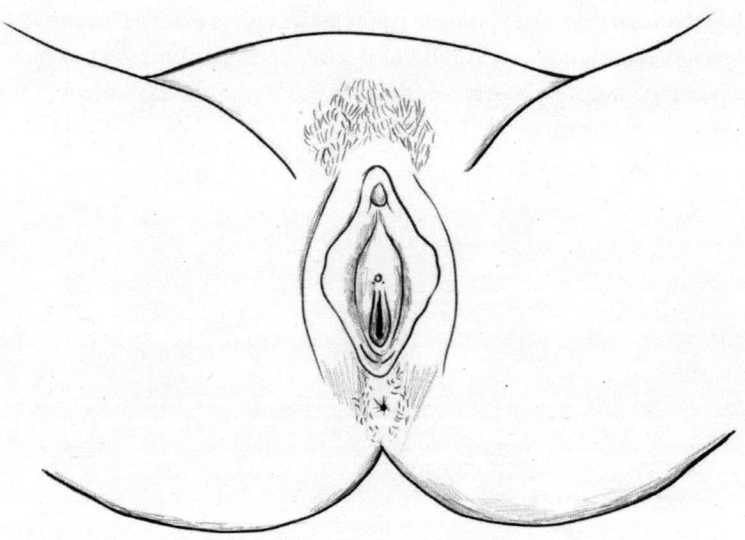

The female external genitalia

Chapter 3

FEMALE HEALTH HORRORS

SHE'S WEARING A DARK RED SUIT, heels, and carries an expensive handbag. As she sits down across from me, a medical student under supervision by a male doctor on a shift in A&E, I can see she's upset. The tears tracking down her face cause her mascara to bleed from her eyelashes and across her cheeks. The doctor puts a hand on her shoulder and gently nudges a box of tissues in her direction.

In that moment, like all medical students when things get serious, I feel as if I'm in the way. I grab my bag and prepare to head for the exit. In response, and without a word, the doctor makes it clear I should remain. I'm glad he did, for what followed was my first step towards enlightenment about women's health.

'I've got some concerns about my . . . ,' she said hesitantly. 'You know . . . down below. My lady bits.'

The patient was in her early forties. Based on her symptoms, the doctor suspected she was going through perimenopause (which we'll get on to later). In that moment the only real certainty was the patient's embarrassment at naming parts of the female anatomy. Every time *vulva*, *vagina*, *clitoris* and *labia* were mentioned in the doctor's assessment that followed, she winced as if such words were meant to be censored.

Eventually, after some gentle probing questions, the patient revealed she had vaginal dryness and a decrease in her libido, both symptoms of perimenopause.

For me, this wasn't the first time that a sense of awkwardness about a health concern had become an obstacle in assessing a patient. In some cases, in fact, it wasn't the patient who struggled but the medical professional, and in many cases it centred around women's health.

Among many other reasons, the sexualisation of women's bodies perpetuates the taboo and stigma around female health. Ultimately this can prevent women getting the medical advice and help they need and, when they do see a doctor, euphemisms are often used to describe their body parts, which risks infantilising and confusing serious medical conditions.

I believe that opening up conversations about difficult health topics starts with language – words can shift our perceptions and change attitudes. And yet even the medical terms for certain parts of women's anatomy are loaded with embarrassment. The word 'pudenda', for example, is used to describe the external genitalia. The Latin root of this word, 'pudere', literally means 'to shame'. Similarly, the word 'clitoris', the vulva's most erogenous area, is derived from the Ancient Greek word meaning 'to sheath, shut or hide'.

This stigma and censorship over female bodies extends to online spaces. Whenever I make social media content about women's health, it's often immediately flagged as inappropriate or potentially pornographic. As a result, my bid to inform and educate is blocked and the taboo or mystery surrounding the subject is reinforced.

I have a mother, a wife, female friends and work colleagues, and maybe one day a daughter. So is it wrong to want them to live in a world where we can openly have these conversations? In school biology lessons, other than a cursory overview of menstruation, we didn't cover female anatomy and I left knowing very little about periods or the actual biology of menstruation.

Surely, I thought, it would get better at medical school, especially as many of my peers were destined to become obstetricians, gynaecologists, endocrinologists or GPs dealing with women's health on a daily basis? Unfortunately, that was a no also. Bar the basic diseases and anatomy, we were taught relatively little about women's health and much of what I know now is down to my own research or clinical experience.

I'm not here to 'mansplain' – except that, well, I am a man – but rather to share what I've learned over the years. This is the stuff that I wish I had known earlier in my career and which I hope will help to destigmatise the range of issues that affect women the world over.

My hope also is that the following pages will help you to disregard many of the bizarre TikTok videos that claim gelatin and flavoured fizzy drinks can help reduce menstrual bleeding or that steaming a vagina like dim sum can relieve cramps.

Instead, here's a basic primer on the 'mystical' world (many would have you believe) of female health.

Vagina or vulva?

Before we begin, it's worth addressing the anatomical elephant in the room and ensure that we all know what we're talking about. The vagina doesn't comprise the entire genital tract. People often use this word to describe female genitalia as though it is the only piece of biology that exists down there. The truth is, female anatomy is wonderfully complex and intricate, so it deserves a proper language to go with it. Vagina is not a catch-all term.

The outside part that you can see and where the skin touches your underwear is called the vulva, not the vagina. The vagina is on the inside. The worlds of the vagina and vulva intersect at the point known as the vestibule of the vaginal opening.

The vulva is histologically (at microscopic cell level) similar to other parts of your skin. It has hair, sweat glands, sebum-producing glands, and is keratinised, meaning it has an outer layer of dead skin cells that are loaded with keratin protein to give you a waterproof protection against the elements.

As you gradually pull back the curtains and traverse deeper, you will pass the labia major and minor until you reach the vagina, a muscular tube connected to your uterus. Here you will find an entire zoo of microbes, the bulk of which will be a bacterial army responsible for vaginal health.

The vagina is alive

You may have come across the phrase that the 'vagina is a self-cleaning oven'. That isn't a cue for people to stick bakery products in there but simply alludes to the fact that the vagina consists of an intricate, delicate ecosystem. It's home to beneficial bacteria like lactobacilli, among others, mucus, viruses, various fungi, yeasts and more. These flora are part of the vaginal microbiome.

This ecosystem works around the clock to keep things 'clean' and maintain an acidic pH in the vagina – yes, the vagina has its own dedicated pH somewhere around 3.8–4.5 to maintain an environment that would be hostile to would-be pathogenic invaders. On a public service note, the normal discharge seen on underwear is a sign this system is working fine to keep pathogens at bay.

The vagina has a degree of 'plasticity', in that it can look after itself. It can recalibrate for slight disruptions in the microbiome (during sex or menstruation, for example) and correct itself. Indeed, there are some vaginal microbiome 'hacks' that have a grounding in science, such as using a menstrual cup to collect and contain blood from a higher region in the vagina so it doesn't fester for long periods of time. Using barrier protection (either a condom or femidom) during the first few weeks of intercourse with a new partner can also limit the influence external microbes can have on the native vaginal flora. A gut-friendly diet can even have a positive effect on the vaginal biome, which means eating fermented and fibre-rich foods like kefir, kombucha, sauerkraut, live yoghurt, fruit and vegetables.

Female health horrors

> ## *The truth about feminine hygiene washes*
>
> Put simply, they're a scam.
>
> A gentle cleanser is OK but most hygiene washes will raise the pH and disrupt the natural acid mantle of the vagina's skin. This could lead to irritation, discharge and odour (which is probably why you tried the product in the first place). Avoid probiotic-enriched cleaning products or supplements for vaginal or vulva health; despite the overwhelming resources of a fraudulent industry, these quasi-scientific chemicals will actually do you harm, while draining your bank balance. Until we have consistent, high-quality evidence for targeted vaginal microbiome products, they are more hype than health.
>
> The problem with these products goes beyond their pseudoscience – they have shifted the mass social belief and distorted the self-perception of countless women. We are being trained to think that vaginas are designed to be fresh and odourless and that our bodies need to constantly be fragrant, like a field of lavender in the height of summer.
>
> The fact is none of us would be here without this extraordinary bit of equipment. Rather than peddling the myth that they somehow 'stink', it's high time we give them the respect they deserve.

Let's talk periods

Periods, or menstruation, are a unique biological phenomenon among mammals. Only humans, ten primate species, four bat species, the elephant shrew and one known species of the spiny mouse menstruate. It's a very selective club to be in.

Menstruation involves the coordination of the brain, ovaries and uterus. The brain pokes the ovaries into action via neurohormonal signals to produce an egg, which leads to a rise in oestrogen and progesterone, and a thickening of the uterine lining to make it hospitable for a possible baby. If there's no pregnancy, however, the lining comes loose resulting in a period.

This Is Vital Information

It is a little more complex than that – so let's delve into the details a little more.

Go with the flow

The first stop in the monthly cycle is the follicular phase. As the leading ovarian follicle (a tiny sac in the ovary) develops, it produces more estradiol, which leads to a rise in oestrogen levels. This tells the lining of the uterus (the endometrium) to thicken and sprout a network of tiny blood vessels in preparation for a potential pregnancy.

During ovulation, the remaining sac of tissue in the ovary transforms into the corpus luteum, a magical, short-lived group of cells that appear once a month to act as a little progesterone-producing factory. This burst of progesterone in turn gets the lining of the uterus ready and geared up for the potential fertilisation of an egg.

If the corpus luteum doesn't get the green light that fertilisation has happened – i.e., there is no pregnancy – the progesterone factory shuts down. This triggers the blood vessels supplying the uterus to spasm and release pro-inflammatory compounds, which eventually causes the top layer of the uterine lining to separate and break down.

And this is what comes out of a woman's body during a period: blood from the broken blood vessels; which you might be surprised to learn makes up only half of menstrual discharge, the rest consisting of fragments of the uterine lining, mucus and inflammatory fluid. As it makes its exit it picks up hitchhikers from the vagina and cervix in the form of cervical mucus and vaginal discharge.

The blood sacrifice

With euphemistic descriptions like 'shark week', some (men) may be tempted to think that women experience a major haemorrhage once a month. But how much blood and discharge is actually produced?

Each menstrual cycle usually sees an average blood loss of 35–50ml and an abnormally heavy flow is defined as blood loss greater than 80–90ml.

Remember, this is only the blood part, so there might be double the amount of fluid in total.

I understand that it's not exactly easy to measure blood flow – I don't expect women to be decanting menstrual blood on to a kitchen weighing scale. If your period is so heavy or painful that it affects the quality of your life then you need to consult a doctor. Menorrhagia, or very heavy menstrual bleeding, is often ignored or undertreated, and could result in iron deficiency or anaemia. Shockingly, 40 per cent of females between the ages of twelve and twenty-one, and almost 20 per cent of those between fourteen and fifty are iron deficient, mostly due to heavy menstrual bleeding.

The following might indicate an abnormal or heavy flow:

- The appearance of large blood clots bigger than 2cm
- Seeping through on to bedding or clothes despite the use of menstrual products
- Excessive changing of tampons or sanitary pads every two hours or more frequently
- Using more than one menstrual product at a time.

International periods

Strawberry week (*erdbeerwoche*), cooking black pudding (*faire du boudin*), the aunt is here (*sono arrivati la zia*), the vampire (*el vampiro*) . . . around the world there are thousands of euphemisms for the word 'period' and I'll admit I'm as guilty as anyone when it comes to euphemisms.

Such linguistic variety often reflects how menstruation and periods are viewed in different cultures. For example, in Sri Lanka a girl may have a 'poopunitha neerattu vizha' at her first menstruation; a party to celebrate a coming of age, equivalent to a sweet sixteen. For others, fate isn't so kind. Many young girls and women never have anything explained to them, such is the taboo and even shame associated with menstruation.

This Is Vital Information

Despite menstruation being so commonplace – I mean *only* 50 per cent of the population experiences it – there is an inordinate amount of stigma that surrounds it. It is, of course, a perfectly natural and healthy part of a woman's reproductive health and while some women breeze through their periods without any issues, many don't and suffer a host of side effects and problems. Some of these might sound unpleasant, strange or bizarre but they are a common experience for women and girls. It's only by bringing discussion of menstruation out in the open that we break through the taboos and empower women to take a greater ownership of their own health.

Cramp corner

Painful cramps during periods are all too common, but what causes them? Well, you can blame prostaglandins, hormone-like substances that contract the muscular layer of the uterus. This causes the blood vessels to become compressed, resulting in a temporary decrease in the supply of oxygen and nutrients to the uterine tissue. Ultimately, this culminates in ischaemia, one of the most painful biological events that can occur in the human body and seen in heart attacks, blood clots in the lung, and labour.

In fact, the pressure generated in the uterus during menstruation can reach 120mmHg, with up to four contractions every ten minutes. That's equivalent to the pressure generated during the second stage of labour (the pushing bit!).

As if this wasn't enough, the prostaglandins can also cause contractions in other tissues beyond the uterus, including the bladder and the bowels. This can lead to a host of 'fun' symptoms, which we'll touch on later. As if that wasn't enough, prostaglandins are also algesic substances (opposite to analgesic pain relievers) in that they heighten pain sensations in the nervous system. This double whammy results in intense and more frequent contractions, with an abnormal rhythm and exponentially exquisite pain.

To reduce the symptoms of cramps, you could try the following:

- Take an NSAID (a non-steroidal anti-inflammatory drug) like ibuprofen just before your period starts (easier for some than others) and for the following couple of days. Ibuprofen works by reducing the production of prostaglandin, reducing pain for up to 80 per cent of women and reducing menstrual flow by up to 40 per cent. (If you have asthma, stomach ulcers, kidney disease or other issues that advise against ibuprofen, consult with your doctor first.)

- Heat can relax muscles and improve blood flow so have a warm bath or put a hot water bottle on your lower stomach. (Be careful of burns and the chronic use of hot water bottles on bare skin as this can lead to skin changes known as erythema ab igne, a potential sign that there is some chronic pain, which should be investigated.)

- Gentle exercise, like walking, swimming or yoga, can also relieve cramps by releasing endorphins.

- Use a TENS (transcutaneous electrical nerve stimulation) machine, which sends electrical impulses to muscles and nerves, blocking and suppressing pain signals to the brain in the process. Place it where you feel pain and see if it provides you with relief.

- Use hormonal contraception, which can help to thin the lining of the uterus, reducing the total amount of prostaglandin produced, resulting in less blood and fewer contractions.

- If your period pain does not get better or worsens, talk to your doctor, who might suggest an ultrasound scan (or other investigations) to check for conditions such as fibroids that can cause heavy periods.

Period pees and poops

If your body turns into a colon sausage churning factory in the midst of your period, don't worry, you are not alone. It happens to at least 28 per cent of women and symptoms can range from bloating and abdominal pain to faecal urgency, diarrhoea and the sensation of incomplete emptying. It's also not uncommon for women to find themselves needing to urinate with increasing frequency during menstruation.

Prostaglandin is mainly responsible for all of the above, along with the hormone progesterone. During the early part of menstruation, progesterone is still lurking in the background, biding its time. At this point your bowel movements are predictable, your bloating is minimal, and your intestines quietly hum along like a well-oiled machine. Enjoy it while it lasts.

Then comes the 'luteal phase', when progesterone makes its grand entrance like an overly enthusiastic party crasher. While it is primarily tasked with preparing the uterine lining for potential pregnancy, it can decide also to have a chat with your intestines. The result? Slower digestive function and intestinal motility, leading to constipation.

Your intestines transform into a stagnant swamp and that salad you ate two days ago is still hanging out, fermenting like it's auditioning for a wine barrel. The slowed motility traps air in your gut, leading to bloating. Add the occasional progesterone-induced craving for chocolate or salty snacks, and your digestive system becomes a ticking time bomb.

As progesterone levels drop, your intestines suddenly wake up, realising they've been slacking for days. Your colon (which is part of the large intestine), drunk on new-found freedom, decides it's time to evacuate everything at once.

This isn't your average bathroom trip, rather it's a full-scale evacuation drill. You might think: 'Did I accidentally drink a gallon of coffee?' No, that's just progesterone's parting gift. Prostaglandins, those mischievous inflammatory chemicals released alongside the hormone drop, however, also irritate the bowels and subsequent progesterone fluctuations turn your colon into an unpredictable roommate – one day calm and quiet, the next throwing wild tantrums. It's the hormone's way of saying: 'I'm busy prepping the uterus, but let's not forget about the intestines – I have anarchy to spread.'

Female health horrors

So the next time you're dealing with pre-period constipation, bloating, or diarrhoea, just remember: your colon isn't lazy, it's just been taken hostage by frenzied hormones. And, unlike most bad guests, these ones happily show up every single month.

A pain in the backside

Just in case bowel discomfort, bleeding, cramps and hormonal mood swings weren't enough – a lucky few women are blessed with an extra special period by-product: proctalgia fugax. Quite literally, this is Latin for fleeting anal pain.

You might be carrying on with your day as normal and then be struck by a lightning bolt in your derrière as if cursed by Zeus himself. This bum-based brutality can occur when the walls of the rectum, anal sphincters and pelvic floor muscles go into spasm. There can be a number of things that trigger proctalgia fugax (meaning that it isn't exclusive to women during periods) but it is more common during menstruation.

Ways to avoid butt pain

Although there's no guaranteed way to rid yourself of proctalgia fugax, there are some things you can try to lessen the symptoms or at least significantly reduce the chances of getting it in the first place:

- Ensure the pain isn't caused by an underlying condition that can be treated and cured. Rectal/anal pain can be a manifestation of common things like haemorrhoids, anal fissures, fistulas or abscesses.

- Keep your derrière clean. Poor peri-anal hygiene and the presence of faecal residue – aka poo flakes – in those forbidden nooks and crannies could trigger an itchy, painful bout of pruritus ani (itchy anus).

- Avoid constipation as this can lead to straining when defecating, which can put undue strain on pelvic floor muscles and the anal area, triggering spasms.

This Is Vital Information

- Go for a walk. A quick way to reduce cramping is movement. Improving blood flow to the area by gentle walking can make a difference on a particularly crampy day.

- Soak in a warm bath or apply warm compresses to help the sphincter muscles to relax.

- Take NSAIDs like ibuprofen as soon as your period starts or the day before if possible. These medications work to reduce the production of prostaglandins and so can help in easing cramps.

- Discuss with your pharmacist or doctor about the potential use of topical creams such as diltiazem or GTN, which can help reverse the spasm and improve blood flow to the area. (Be careful if you are on blood pressure medications as these could drop your blood pressure.)

- Yoga and other simple stretches can help to relax tight pelvic floor muscles. One useful exercise involves lying on your back with both knees bent and your feet touching the ground. Bring your knees towards your shoulders and hold for three seconds.

Mystery pain

It's 8am. I've just started a thirteen-hour shift when I get a referral from A&E.

'We have a 21-year-old woman with a three-day history of severe lower abdominal pain, negative pregnancy test and urine, normal blood tests. Could you review to rule out appendicitis?'

I assess the patient. She's in excruciating pain and yet her history and examination doesn't fit with appendicitis or any obvious surgical pathology. I prescribe pain relief and organise a pelvic and abdominal ultrasound to exclude any obvious gynaecological issue.

The ultrasound comes back clear and the young woman is reviewed by the consultant (my boss at the time). He explains to her that because her blood tests and scans are normal, she will be discharged and that her pain is 'probably period-related'.

Female health horrors

The patient returns the same night with worse pain. The overnight doctor organises a CT scan. This is also normal. From there, we contact the gynaecology team to assess her. Suspecting a diagnosis of a 'ruptured ovarian cyst', they reassure the patient that this is very common and discharge her.

The patient returns two days later. She's still in agony. It's a new consultant on call and I ask if it's worth investigating this pain with a more invasive test: a diagnostic laparoscopy, a minimally invasive surgery that involves placing a telescopic camera inside the abdomen. After much pestering, my boss relents and allows me to take the patient to theatre.

Before you assume that this is the work of an eager-to-operate surgeon, I must inform you that surgeons actually don't 'like' to operate. It should be the last resort. A former boss once told me: 'A good surgeon can operate, a better surgeon knows *when* to operate, but the best surgeons know when *not* to operate.'

With this aphorism swirling through my mind, along with the repeated trips to the hospital endured by this young woman, I believed we had reached the final stop: surgery.

As I inserted the laparoscope and assessed the abdominal and pelvic cavity, I noticed dark patches like plaques on the patient's uterus and ovaries. Immediately, I called the gynaecologists to the operating room for a second opinion. They confirmed what I had feared, and it proved to be a life-changing diagnosis: endometriosis.

Everything about endometriosis

Endometriosis is a chronic condition in which tissue similar to the lining of the uterus grows in other sites such as the pelvic cavity, fallopian tubes and ovaries. Endometrioid tissue has even been found on the bladder, the intestines and in rare cases as far away as the diaphragm, lungs and brain. Untreated, it can cause infertility and generally ruin lives.

Endometriosis isn't just a disease of misplaced uterine tissue; it's a stark metaphor for how the medical system often misplaces its priorities when it comes to women's health. We insist on pigeonholing diseases like endometriosis into narrow, gynaecological categories. If it doesn't disrupt the reproductive system, it's dismissed as irrelevant. But this is medical myopia. Endometriosis is not just a 'woman's problem'; it's a systemic condition capable of disrupting nearly every bodily system. The plaques and lesions can invade pelvic nerves, inflame the peritoneum (the inner lining of the abdominal cavity), distort bowel function, and even travel as far as the diaphragm to cause chest pain, shortness of breath and even haemoptysis (coughing up blood). In fact, there has been at least one case report in the medical literature of endometriosis found in . . . the eye!

Though not typical, it isn't rare – it's estimated that up to 10 per cent of ovulating women have endometriosis and it can take ten years on average to get a diagnosis. Even worse, we don't know about the causes or why some women are more likely to get it. It's also one of those subjects people don't know or like to talk about. Period cramps? Poor you.

The medical community is also guilty of disregarding the debilitating effects of endometriosis – pain is 'expected' during periods – resulting in a distinct lack of focus, education and study into this chronic condition.

Thinking back over my medical career, both undergraduate and postgraduate, it started to make sense. There was a deep lack of understanding of gynaecological health, and I don't excuse myself from this cohort. It wasn't something extensively covered in medical school, bar the basic diseases and anatomy. In my experience, there seemed to be an institutional disregard for the potential of chronic female health conditions to be debilitating, a normalisation of high thresholds of pain that is 'expected' during periods and ultimately a failure of the medical community to do further research in women's health. In this view, my sincerest hope is that in some small way, this chapter contributes something towards positive change. And maybe, just maybe, we'll begin dismantling the entrenched biases that have kept women waiting far too long for answers.

Female health horrors

What should you do if you suspect you have endometriosis?

- **Recognise the signs:** Endometriosis is a condition that can present with a constellation of symptoms, some of which might seem unrelated to gynaecology. Classic symptoms include: chronic pelvic pain, often worse during menstruation, excessively heavy or irregular periods, painful sex (dyspareunia), infertility or difficulty conceiving.

- **Keep a symptom diary:** Document pain, bleeding and other symptoms (e.g., digestive or musculoskeletal issues) to present a comprehensive picture to your doctor.

- **Demand a thorough investigation:** Seek referrals to gynaecologists who specialise in endometriosis. Request a discussion regarding diagnostic imaging such as pelvic ultrasounds or an MRI, although note these may not detect all cases. Request a discussion about the role of laparoscopy if symptoms are severe, as it remains the gold standard for diagnosis (according to the National Institute for Health and Care Excellence, or NICE, guidelines at the time of writing).

- **Challenge a dismissal:** If a doctor downplays your pain or symptoms, don't hesitate to seek a second opinion. Women are often conditioned to endure pain as 'normal', but chronic pain isn't normal.

- **Educate yourself:** Read trusted resources on endometriosis to understand its systemic nature. Online forums in which people exchange anecdotes and personal experiences are often deeply validating and helpful in navigating your own journey.

Press pause

What if I told you there's a condition leading to an increased risk of heart disease, dementia and early death? It's one that has affected humans for as long as we have existed. The host of symptoms can be very unpleasant, ranging from headaches and memory problems to anxiety and weight gain.

This Is Vital Information

What if I then added that over half the world's population suffer from this condition at some point in their life. You might assume it would be a constant topic of conversation, studied by many of the world's leading scientists and a topic taught in schools. If so, you would be wrong.

The condition I'm talking about is menopause (and perimenopause) and it affects 1.2 billion women worldwide. It's not a disease but its impact can be profound.

The medical definition of menopause is pretty clear-cut: it is a phase in a woman's life marked by the end of menstrual periods due to reduced ovarian function. A female is born with more than a million eggs nestled away safely in the ovaries. Every month (give or take), one is released. The release of eggs is facilitated by the hormone oestrogen, which is involved in a significant number of crucial bodily functions: brain health, breast development, bone density, reproductive health, bowel function, fat deposition and storage, and beyond.

The perimenopause is the time when a woman's body makes a gradual transition towards menopause, combined with lower levels of oestrogen production, which can happen over several months or years. Menopause usually hits around the age of fifty-one years but around one in a hundred, probably more, women under the age of forty have an early menopause and run out of eggs a bit earlier. This might be because they had a low baseline of eggs in the first place, had their ovaries removed from surgery, or their ovaries were damaged by taking medication or as a result of chemotherapy or radiotherapy.

For a long time menopause was considered a time of transition that would last a few years, cause a few hot flushes and then it was over and done with. It is true that about 20 per cent of women will have few or no symptoms, but we also know that about 25 per cent of women have severe symptoms that seriously impact their lives.

These symptoms can range from inconvenient to existentially unsettling, including vaginal dryness, mood swings, cognitive impairment known as 'brain fog', abnormal bowel symptoms, joint issues, skin changes, sleep abnormalities, and a bone density decline that makes you wonder if your skeleton has a grudge against you. The tissues lining the vagina can also become thin and less stretchy, which can lead to pain and discomfort during penetrative sex and when sitting down for long periods.

> ### Mansplaining the menopause
>
> As a doctor who is not a gynaecologist and not female (despite many of those seeing my name as Karen not Karan), I like to rationalise the complex world of women's health for my very simple surgical and male brain.
>
> So here are some things it's worth *everyone* knowing about the menopause:
>
> - **It's a marathon not a sprint:** Menopause marks the finishing line of the great ovulation race. Most of the oestrogen in women is produced by the developing eggs within the ovaries. So it stands to reason that when these ovarian follicles can no longer produce the same amount of oestrogen to trigger menstruation, the body will mark the occasion. Hello menopause.
>
> - **Reverse puberty rollercoaster:** OK, so menopause is not puberty (obviously) but there are some mirroring features. The symptoms leading up to menopause – the perimenopause – can often be worse than menopause itself due to the wild fluctuations of hormone bingo that happens – think sleep disturbances, hot flushes and so on – which in some cases can be a rude reminder of your teenage angst.
>
> - **The one-year anniversary:** While it might not be something to celebrate, medically speaking, one year on from the last menstrual period is a marker that you're officially part of the menopause club. Congratulations is not required, you've paid your dues, you've earned this membership.

- **Menopause is not a disease:** It is a commonly held belief that menopause is a state of hormone deficiency. This implies that, like nutrient or hormone deficiencies in other conditions (think low thyroxine and hypothyroidism), menopause is a disease. This is wrong. Instead, it is a normal physiological phase of life and a simple consequence of ageing. We don't define girls before puberty as deficient in oestrogen, so why should menopausal women succumb to this label?

- **You are not losing your mind:** Brain fog in menopause is a common occurrence, but it is not a marker of cognitive decline. In most cases, it's a temporary not permanent change to memory and cognition.

- **Menopause can be associated with other diseases:** Menopause can certainly increase the *risk* (key word) of conditions like neurodegeneration, cardiovascular disease and osteoporosis. The longer someone goes through menopause, the greater the risk. Being armed with this knowledge means you can take steps to prevent these diseases (think diet, exercise, optimising sleep, etc.).

- **Hormonal treatment isn't a holy grail:** While some might herald hormone therapy as a panacea for every menopause symptom, or vital for every single woman, this is untrue and does not align with menopause guidelines or science. Oestrogen can help with some symptoms like hot flushes, sleep issues and mood (in some cases) and certainly in helping to reduce the risk of osteoporosis, but it isn't a one-size-fits-all solution.

HORMONES

Menopause is having a moment, from documentaries about it to celebrities opening up about their experiences and online communities bringing forth more information about perimenopause and menopause.

Female health horrors

You would think that bringing the discussion about menopause out in the open could only be a good thing. But there are still lots of gaps in our understanding, which unscrupulous influencers like to fill with dodgy claims, drowning out the noise of the legitimate conversations about the topic.

The sad truth is, false claims about menopause hormones, scam-ridden supplements from celebrity influencers and doctors, the promotion of dodgy menopause diets and tests have flooded the halls of misinformation.

Let's dial in on the misinformation about menopause hormone therapy (MHT), previously known as HRT (hormone replacement therapy), and the far-fetched claims that have infected the internet. MHT has been positioned as the fountain of youth that can reduce a person's risk of dementia and cardiovascular disease, and is thus essential for every woman reaching this point in their life. The sales pitch is fear-based, making it rife for manipulation by social media algorithms.

MHT is the hormonal equivalent of calling in reinforcements when menopause decides to turn your body into its personal battlefield. Essentially, it's a treatment that supplements the oestrogen and sometimes progesterone that your ovaries have decided they're done producing, like a bartender cutting you off after decades of hormonal happy hours.

Given the long list of horrible perimenopause and menopause symptoms, it is no surprise that women would want to see some of these side effects banished with a simple act of taking MHT. But does everyone really need it? MHT absolutely improves the quality of life for those who require it and if a woman is at risk of osteoporosis, it can also be beneficial. Currently, however, we don't have irrefutable data to support the claim that MHT reduces the risk of dementia or cardiovascular disease, although research is ongoing.

On the other side of the coin, some sceptics have claimed that MHT is an inherently dangerous treatment, which has proven equally damaging. The risks of blood clots and breast cancer associated with MHT have often been exaggerated due to a misinterpretation of studies. This has caused a reluctance among some people to take MHT, despite its potential benefits.

The study that fuelled the myth

The Women's Health Initiative (WHI) was a landmark study that looked at the effects of MHT on women's health. For those taking MHT, it reported increased risks of breast cancer, heart disease and blood clots, which dramatically shifted public perception about MHT. However, its findings have since been re-evaluated due to several issues. The study included women with an average age of sixty-three, many of whom were already years past menopause and not reflective of the typical demographic of women starting MHT in their forties or fifties. Moreover, many participants had pre-existing health conditions, skewing the results.

The WHI study reported a 26 per cent relative increase in breast cancer risk for women using combined oestrogen–progestin therapy. But this translated to an increase of only four additional cases per 1,000 women over five years. In other words, the vast majority of women did not develop breast cancer.

The risk of blood clots (deep vein thrombosis or pulmonary embolism) was also exaggerated. While there is a small increase in risk, taking oral contraceptives or a long-haul flight have similar risk factors.

The increased risk of blood clots with oral MHT is about one additional case per 1,000 women annually. Transdermal oestrogen, delivered via patches, gels or spray, carries negligible risk since it bypasses the liver.

Despite risks, WHI studies showed MHT could reduce certain cancers. Combined MHT may lower colorectal cancer risk by up to 40 per cent, and when paired with progesterone, it protects against endometrial cancer, a risk for women on oestrogen-only therapy with intact uteruses.

It is important to consider these statistics in the context of the general risks women face for certain conditions after menopause as they age.

For instance, one in two women over the age of fifty who don't take MHT will develop osteoporosis, a loss of bone density, and of those, one in three will have an osteoporotic hip fracture. Additionally, a woman's risk of a heart attack increases five-fold after menopause due to a decline in oestrogen, a hormone that protects the heart and blood vessels.

Other tools

If you decide MHT isn't for you, don't despair. There are lots of simple, non-invasive steps that could help alleviate the symptoms of menopause.

1. Sleep and menopause

Sleep disturbances, including insomnia and fragmented sleep, are common during menopause. Oestrogen loss impacts the hypothalamus – a small, vital area in the brain that affects certain body functions – which disrupts the regulation of body temperature, leading to night sweats. At the same time, progesterone, a natural sedative, also declines, affecting sleep quality and increasing wakefulness. To help with sleep issues during menopause:

- **Optimise sleep hygiene**
  - Maintain a consistent sleep schedule.
  - Create a dark, cool bedroom environment.
  - Avoid screens an hour before bed as blue light suppresses melatonin.

- **Try cognitive behavioural therapy for insomnia (CBT-I)**
  - Several studies have found CBT-I to be effective for improving sleep quality in menopausal women.

- **Take supplements**
  - **Melatonin:** This could help regulate sleep–wake cycles disrupted by menopause (1–3mg). Consult with your doctor before taking it and this should not be viewed as a quick fix.

- o **Magnesium:** Some evidence suggests it may support muscle relaxation and thus potentially calm the nervous system.
- **Limit triggers**
  - o Avoid caffeine and alcohol close to bedtime; both can disrupt sleep and exacerbate hot flushes.

2. Gut health and diet

Oestrogen loss during menopause can lead to an imbalance or disruption of the gut's microbiome, known as dysbiosis. This can cause a wide range of symptoms, including bloating, constipation, changes in bowel habits, inflammation, fatigue, worsening other menopausal symptoms. Here's how to avoid dysbiosis and support a healthy microbiome.

- **Increase your intake of prebiotic foods**, which feed beneficial gut bacteria, promote diversity, reduce inflammation and support the gut lining.
  - o Top prebiotic foods include garlic, onions, leeks, asparagus, green bananas and whole grains, like oats and barley.
- **Include probiotics** in your diet like lactobacillus and bifidobacterium strains, which can help modulate the microbiome and reduce symptoms like bloating and constipation.
  - o Typical probiotics include yoghurt with live cultures, kefir, sauerkraut and kimchi.
- **Eat foods rich in polyphenols**, which enhance beneficial bacteria and reduce gut inflammation.
  - o **Foods rich in polyphenols include** berries, green tea, dark chocolate, nuts, seeds and spices.
- **Reduce gut irritants**
  - o Limit excessive salt, high quantities of ultra-processed foods, and alcohol, which can disrupt gut bacteria and increase inflammation.

Other tips for a healthy diet during menopause:

- **Focus on plant-based foods** that contain antioxidants and are high in fibre.
    - Foods include lentils, chickpeas, flaxseeds and soy products.
- **Prioritise protein**, which can help mitigate muscle loss and supports metabolism. In the peri- and post-menopause stages, aim for 1.2g/kg/day (potentially higher if engaging in lots of physical activity). A useful formula is your weight (kg) x g/kg/day = daily target (g).
    - Sources include eggs, lean meats, tofu and legumes.
- **East healthy fats:** omega-3 fats reduce inflammation and improve heart health.
    - Typical sources include oily fish, walnuts and chia seeds.
- **Ensure your diet includes calcium and vitamin D**, which support bone health and reduce fracture risk.
    - Typical sources: milk, cheese, yoghurt, fortified plant milk, leafy greens.

3. Skincare and menopause

Oestrogen supports collagen production, skin elasticity, and hydration. Its decline leads to thinner, drier skin, fine lines and wrinkles due to reduced collagen and increased sensitivity and slower wound healing.

- **Use hydrating ingredients**
    - **Hyaluronic acid:** retains water and plumps the skin.
    - **Ceramides:** rebuilds the skin barrier to combat dryness.
- **Retinoids**
    - Stimulate collagen production and reduce wrinkles.
    - Use at night to avoid sensitivity.

Use a gentle cleanser on your skin and moisturise while skin is still damp to lock in moisture.

- **Use sun protection**
    - Oestrogen decline increases susceptibility to UV damage.
    - Use SPF 30+ daily and reapply when needed.
- **Keep hydrated and have a healthy diet**
    - Stay hydrated and consume omega-3s (flaxseeds, walnuts, salmon) to maintain skin elasticity.

4. Physical activity and menopause

Menopause accelerates bone density loss and muscle loss and increases cardiovascular risk. Regular exercise mitigates these effects and improves mood, sleep and cardiovascular health. Types of exercise to try include:

- **Weight-bearing exercises**, such as walking, jogging or dancing, which stimulate bone remodelling and reduces the risk of osteoporosis.
- **Resistance training** to build muscle and improve metabolism.
- **Aerobic exercise**, such as cycling, swimming or walking, reduces blood pressure, cholesterol and inflammation.
- **Yoga, pilates and stretching** alleviate joint stiffness, improve flexibility and reduce stress.

BREAST HEALTH

It's darkly ironic that while breasts have been the centre of cultural obsession for millennia, we barely talk about them in a meaningful way. From Renaissance paintings that made them divine symbols of virtue and fertility, to modern ad campaigns where they're pixelated and censored like state secrets, the conversation hasn't exactly evolved.

What people are really talking about is rarely breast *health*. Instead, it's the idea of breasts: too big, too small, too visible, too saggy, too uncovered.

And somewhere in the noise, the fact that they're an actual, functional part of a woman's anatomy capable of nourishing life, sending cancer alarms, or just existing as part of a body gets completely lost.

Even now, as I write this, there's undoubtedly someone somewhere enraged at the sight of a mother breastfeeding in public, decrying it as 'indecent'. Meanwhile, society is busy raking in billions from various industries selling sexualised images of women and their breasts.

Like genitals, breasts have managed to amass a number of nicknames and euphemisms that humanity has lovingly, awkwardly and occasionally offensively bestowed upon them: boobs, knockers, melons, kittens, baps, bazoongas, funbags, bangers, sweater meat (?!), flapjacks, hooters, honkers, sugar bags, coconuts – I could go on.

It's impressive and weird, really. Few other body parts have inspired such creativity, and even fewer have been granted this much airtime in the cultural consciousness. We don't sit around inventing cute or vaguely threatening nicknames for elbows or spleens, do we? But breasts demand attention. They've become both canvas and commodity; admired, shamed and ridiculed in equal measure.

Joking aside, there is a serious note to this conversation and why we need to have it. Around the world breast cancer is the most common cancer, and in the UK and US it is the second most common cause of cancer-related deaths in women after lung cancer. Having worked as a doctor in breast clinics and engaging with followers online, I've realised that so many people want to learn more about breast health but shockingly there seems to be a lack of useful information.

Are my breasts normal?

Yes. No. Maybe. The truth is, there is no 'normal' when it comes to breasts, just a glorious spectrum of shapes, sizes and quirks as unique as the people they belong to. Breasts are less a template and more a personal work of art, sculpted by hormones, time and the occasional betrayal of gravity. So, instead let's embrace the chaotic masterpiece they are.

If you've ever looked in the mirror and thought: 'Why is one bigger than the other?', you're not alone. Asymmetry is the rule, not the exception. One breast might be larger or smaller, sit higher or lower, or have a different shape entirely. In fact, up to a cup size of difference between breasts is completely normal. Your body isn't a machine that is a result of nature churning out perfect duplicates, it's more of a biological jazz improvisation.

Breasts are also shapeshifters, changing size and texture at different life stages. During your menstrual cycle, they may swell or feel lumpier (thanks, hormones). During pregnancy and breastfeeding, they might double as milk factories, and, as you age, they may descend, like loyal companions deciding they've had enough of the high life.

Your nipples are equally unique, coming in various shapes, sizes and colours. Most protrude a few millimetres above the areola (the darker skin surrounding the nipple), but some may be more subtle, blending into the surrounding skin. Around 10 per cent of people have at least one inverted nipple, a perfectly normal variation that doesn't even prevent breastfeeding.

Nipples can be cone-shaped, flat or round, and the areola has its own personality too, varying in size, colour and texture between breasts. And let's not forget the Montgomery tubercles, those tiny bumps around the areola. They're not just decorative; they secrete oils to keep the skin healthy, making your breasts surprisingly self-sufficient little ecosystems.

Breasts can feel lumpy, smooth, or something in between, and all are normal. If your breasts feel like someone tucked frozen peas under the surface, you might have nodular breasts, a common variation, especially if it's symmetrical and consistent. Hormones often stir the pot, making breasts lumpier in the second half of the menstrual cycle as they prepare for your period. It's biology's way of keeping things interesting.

However, any new changes, like a lump, swelling or difference in texture, warrant a chat with your doctor. Think of it as an early warning system, not a panic button.

Here's the thing: nobody else can tell a woman what's normal for her breasts. Regularly examining them is both a health precaution and an act of self-awareness. By familiarising herself with their quirks, the bumps, textures and asymmetries, a woman will know when something feels off. Rather than being led by fear, the focus is on building trust; trusting that your body knows how to alert you when something's wrong, as long as you're paying attention.

How to check your breasts

- **Look:** Stand in front of a mirror. Hands on hips, then arms up. Check for dimpling, swelling, asymmetry, or a nipple going rogue
- **Feel:** Use three fingers and apply firm pressure (not just a light prod). Pick a method:
    o Concentric circles: Start at the nipple, moving outwards in slow, circular motions
    o Quadrant method: Divide your breast into four sections, plus armpit. Check each thoroughly
- **Squeeze:** Any unexplained discharge? If yes, get it checked.

Do this monthly. Changes matter. Lumps aren't always cancer, but the earlier you get them checked out the better.

Breast pain

If you've ever felt an ache, twinge, tenderness or discomfort in your chest and immediately thought 'is this cancer?', let me offer some reassurance: you're not unique in this pang of panic, and it's usually not. In fact, seven out of ten women will experience breast pain (aka mastalgia) at some point and, for the vast majority, it's mild and manageable.

For most women, breast pain is like a particularly whiny co-worker. It's annoying but not something you'd quit over. Often, the real culprit is your menstrual cycle, with oestrogen and progesterone wreaking their predictable havoc on breast tissue.

Around one in ten women, however, experience moderate to severe breast pain that goes beyond nuisance territory. If you're in this unlucky percentile, you're not imagining it. Keeping a pain diary for a few months, tracking when the pain occurs and its intensity, can help you identify if it's cyclical (linked to your period) or not. If nothing else, keeping a boob journal can make for an excellent conversation starter.

Pain vs panic: the breast cancer fear

Here's the part where we address the 'awkward' topic many people shy away from: breast cancer. It's perfectly natural for your mind to jump to the worst-case scenario when something doesn't feel right; after all, we've been conditioned by decades of public campaigns and internet horror stories. But breast pain alone is rarely a sign of cancer.

Breast cancer typically presents as a painless lump or a thickened area, not as widespread discomfort. Pain that affects both breasts is even less likely to be linked to cancer as your body just isn't that symmetrical when it comes to misery. Of course, if the pain is unusual, persistent, or paired with other symptoms (like a lump, nipple discharge or skin changes), you should absolutely see your doctor. Not because panic is warranted, but because certainty beats sitting at home googling 'weird breast pain' at the crack of dawn.

Pain has a nasty way of hijacking our thoughts. Your brain, ever the pessimist and worrier, often interprets unexplained pain as a harbinger of doom. This isn't your fault. It's evolutionary. Our ancestors had to assume every ache was life-threatening because back then it usually was. Now, though, most pain is just your body's way of saying 'Please pay attention here,' not 'Sound the alarms and prepare for battle.'

The unchangeable realities

Sometimes, cancer has an element of a cosmic dice roll about it and the risk factors can be completely out of your control. No amount of chia seed smoothies or morning yoga can change these.

- **Being born female:** Breasts, it turns out, come with a fine print that includes increased cancer risk. Thanks, evolution.

- **Age:** The older you get, the higher the risk. Your cells, much like your favourite pair of jeans, wear down with time and start making mistakes when dividing.

- **Family history:** The majority of people with breast cancer don't have a family history. But if you do, particularly if a close relative was diagnosed young, your risk increases. Around 5–10 per cent of breast cancers are hereditary, caused by genetic mutations like BRCA1 or BRCA2. If you have one of these mutations, your risk of developing breast cancer can skyrocket to 70 per cent.

- **Dense breast tissue:** If your breasts are more glandular than fatty, you have 'dense breasts'. This not only increases your risk but makes mammograms about as easy to interpret as a blurry photo of Bigfoot.

- **Hormonal exposure:** Starting your period early or hitting menopause late means more lifetime exposure to oestrogen and progesterone. Hormones: great for reproduction, less great for cellular overgrowth.

- **Ethnicity and height:** In the US, breast cancer is more common in white women but often more aggressive in Black women. Taller women have a slightly higher risk of developing breast cancer.

The modifiable factors

Reassuringly, though, there is stuff you can control – not because you're to blame if you get cancer (you're not), but because small changes can make a difference.

- **Weight:**
  - Fat cells don't just sit there; they act like little hormone factories, producing oestrogen and increasing inflammation. Both can raise your risk. Maintaining a healthy weight is easier said than done, but even small steps towards a healthy weight help.

- **Exercise**:
  - Move your body. Walk, dance, lift things . . . whatever gets you moving. An active lifestyle is associated with a lower risk of breast cancer, and it doesn't have to involve running marathons.

- **Alcohol**:
  - Unsurprising at this point, but the more you drink, the higher your risk of breast cancer. Even moderate drinking can nudge the odds up, so if you're a wine-with-dinner kind of person, consider swapping a few glasses for sparkling water.

- **Smoking**:
  - As with most cancers, smoking increases your risk. It's not just your lungs that suffer; tobacco toxins cause issues with breast tissue, too.

I'll level with you: you can do everything 'right' and still get breast cancer. That's not a reason to give up; it's a reason to let go of the illusion of control. Life is messy, unfair and deeply unpredictable, but it's also resilient. Your job isn't to obsess over prevention but to pay attention to your body, examine your breasts regularly, and if something feels off, get it checked. Breast pain, changes in texture or lumps are prompts to see your doctor because early detection matters far more than perfection.

Female health horrors

Mansplaining breasts

Breast cancer is often thought of as an exclusively female domain, but biology doesn't discriminate. Yes, men can and do get breast cancer. Granted, it's far less common (about one in 870 men in the UK will be diagnosed with breast cancer, compared with one in seven women), but the outcomes for men are often worse than for women. Because men, bless our blissful ignorance, rarely think to check their chests for lumps unless someone dares to insult their gym progress.

The problem isn't just biology, it's general awareness – or a lack of it. Most men don't even realise they *have* breast tissue, let alone that it could be a problem for them, and men are far more likely to shrug off warning signs. A lump? Surely nothing more than a stubborn pec muscle. What about this strange discharge? Bah . . . let's ignore it because talking about nipples in public is somehow emasculating, right?

Now, speaking of men . . .

This Is Vital Information

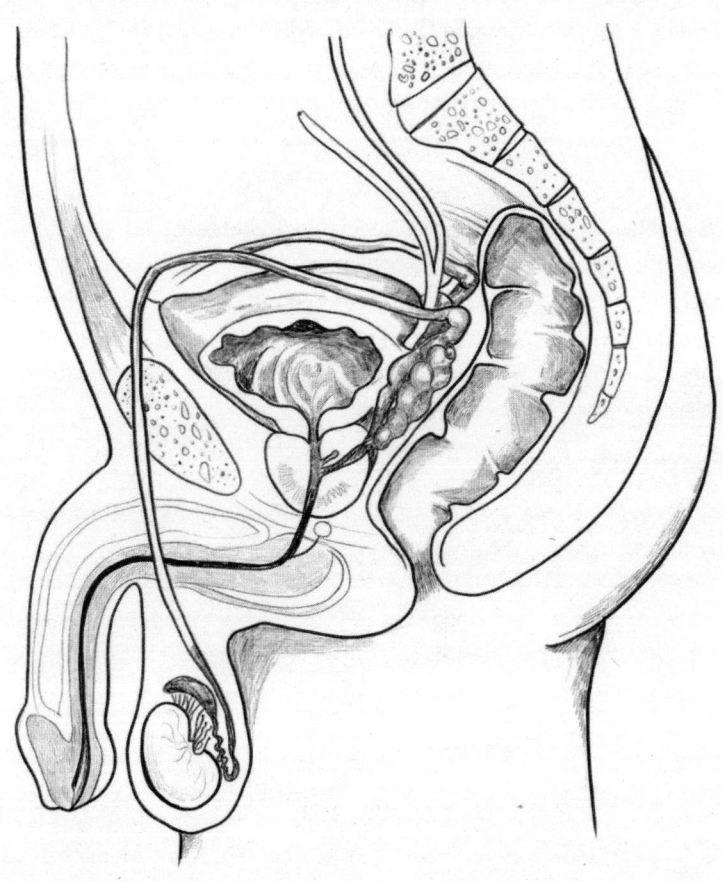

The male reproductive system

Chapter 4

MALE HEALTH HELL

THE PORK SWORD, purple-headed snake, gooey cannon, one-eyed meat cyclops, trouser snake, skin flute, devil's clarinet, schnozwangler, pen15, whangdoodle, meat stick, custard launcher, flesh gherkin, hairy bagpipe, knob, pecker . . . I've used these words and more to describe the male member. The self-proclaimed king of male organs. The penis.

Hearing, seeing or even saying the word 'penis' can seem overly provocative at times, even though it rears its head (see what I did there?) almost everywhere, from aubergine emojis to internet porn and your average *Game of Thrones* scene. There's no doubt that the penis would love to have more airtime, and many owners are all too happy to get it out at the first opportunity. For the vast majority, however, it's an organ that has never quite escaped from the realm of the taboo. Men don't always like to talk openly about their lil' soldier, and consequently that's where myths, uncertainty and anxiety can breed.

I feel sorry for the penis. It often finds itself the butt of jokes. It's also used as an expletive or insult more than in an anatomical sense. It's given a hard time but let me lift back the hood and shed some light on this exquisitely vital and complex structure, which holds the key to pleasure and serves as a window to well-being and a man's health.

This Is Vital Information

A brief history of the penis

The penis has seen and been through it all. At various junctures throughout history, it has been deified, demonised and medicalised in equal measure.

Phallic adoration is not a new phenomenon – ancient cultures were seemingly just as obsessed with the male member as we are today. As an example, Min, the Ancient Egyptian god of fertility, was represented as a human with a large erection. According to many Hindu scholars, the 'lingam', a cylindrical stone with a rounded top, positioned vertically, is suggested to be a phallic symbol (although many Hindus have some discomfort with this interpretation).

Further east, the Shinto religion in Japan has elaborate phallus-filled shrines and an annual 'harvest festival', or Honensai – a fertility ritual that involves the participants parading a giant phallus through the streets.

To the Ancient Greeks, however, massive schlongs were abhorrent, grotesque even. It's thought they considered a small member as a sign of self-control and intelligence and a larger tool as a manifestation of unfiltered, animalistic idiocy and lack of restraint.

Similarly, the Romans, who drew their cultural values heavily from the Greeks, made their statues with diminutive dicks. They even believed large penises were laughable. Take Priapus, a Roman god of fertility. He was basically represented in the form of a large scarecrow with an enormous phallus used to punish people through penetration with his ridiculously oversized piece. In fact, the condition of an extremely painful and prolonged erection is known as priapism, a name derived from the very same god.

Penis size

Size matters. At least it does psychologically for many people. In fact, genital politics and penile grandeur is one of the biggest self-esteem issues men face. With 4 billion penises floating around on planet Earth, anyone hoping to find a true indication of the average penile length faces a gargantuan task.

Thankfully, some rogue scientists had the balls to conduct a census in the name of research. In 2014, they conducted a review based on average penis size data from more than 15,000 men around the world. It's worth noting that the raw data was not based on self-reporting, but from a standard measuring procedure carried out by health professionals.

You're eager to hear the results. You might be surprised. The study revealed that the average length of a flaccid penis was 3.6in (9.16cm) and the average length of an erect penis was 5.165in (13.12cm).

If you're shocked by . . . well, the modest size of those figures, you're unlikely to be alone.

Societal expectations, warped by pornography, Hollywood, rumours and overzealous exaggeration, leave most men thinking the average penis size is closer to something like 6in (15.2cm) or even bigger. Most men regrettably assume they are smaller than average and this distortion fuels a negative self-perception of the body. It can even have a knock-on effect in sexual scenarios.

I'd be surprised if most men hadn't at some point googled the exact sentence 'How do I make my penis bigger?'

This penile 'bigorexia' is so prevalent that it can literally change scientific data. In studies that examined mean penis length based on self-reporting, the average came out at more than an inch larger than studies using *hard* data with tape measures. In a toxic cycle of negative body images, these reports furthered the idea of penile petiteness, effectively exacerbating the problem.

As a keen amateur statistician, I should stress that the average or mean only tells you part of the story. When you look at penis size distribution curves (yes, that's a thing), it turns out that most penises are pretty similar in size, with extreme size discrepancies (very large or very small) being the outliers in the top or bottom 5 per cent. So, 90 per cent of the male population will likely have a penis size around the same number.

Twice as long

If that's not enough reassurance, in further good news, the purple-headed cyclops is twice as long as you think it is.

I've had the blessing (or curse) of examining MRI scans of penises in my time working in urological surgery. There, I can see clearly that half the length of the didgeridoo extends inside the pelvic region and forms a boomerang shape. Unfortunately (or fortunately depending on your persuasion), this isn't visible externally. The root of the penis is fixed to the pubic bone and held in place by the suspensory ligament.

So those opting for 'penis lengthening' surgery, often have this suspensory ligament cut. With the fixation point released, the penis is allowed to flop out more. Unfortunately, this doesn't make your willy wonka any longer; it just makes it hang lower and you lose the angle of your dangle. Not ideal.

Age concern

Like everything else in your body, the crown jewels are affected by age. In this case, they undergo some shrinkage with time. If a man has an erect penis of 6in long in his twenties, it's likely to be 5½in or slightly less beyond the age of sixty.

Besides ageing, carrying extra weight, particularly in the lower abdominal or pubic region, can make the penis appear smaller. There are also certain conditions that can change the shape of the penis. Peyronie's disease is a main contender. This is when a build-up of scar tissue underneath the penile surface can cause excessive curvature when erect.

Age-related conditions like atherosclerosis can also affect arteries supplying the one-eyed snake. This is caused by a build-up of plaque that reduces blood flow and makes the penis appear smaller. Declining testosterone levels that come with age also affects the size and function of the meat and two veg.

The good news is that there are things that can be done to at least slow down the rate of volume loss and bring some extra vitality to this crucially important and boisterous member of the human body.

Bigger, harder, stronger

There is no shortage of charlatans and online sales outlets looking to flog dick-lengthening nutritional supplements or penis pills. Unfortunately, most won't help the biological snake. The published evidence here is limited; if there was a supplement that truly worked on a clinical level to increase penis length, I'd happily bet both my flesh marbles that Big Pharma would have capitalised on this *big* opportunity.

There is limited evidence to show that some natural supplements improve blood flow to the penis or make it transiently plumper, but the studies have often been limited and mired in bias. Quite simply, most products are pulling your leg – just not your third one.

With this in mind, here are a couple of supplements associated with limited studies, with the caveat that there is no guarantee they will increase the penis size in any meaningful way. Many supplements are exorbitantly priced to exploit the self-conscious man hoping to be harder, bigger, or last longer. What's more, some 'herbal' supplements can interact with existing medication and increase their side effects, so you have been warned.

- **Ginseng:** In some studies, the herbal remedy of Korean red ginseng is said to improve erectile dysfunction. The belief is it increases the production of nitric oxide, which acts as fuel for the penis by increasing blood flow (a similar mechanism to how Viagra produces its effects).
- **Horny goat weed:** Just like it says on the tin, this claims to improve sexual function. However, studies are extremely limited

and those that do exist suggest the active ingredient icariin increases the production of nitric oxide.

Ode to the penis

The human penis is a biological masterpiece, equal parts functional, fragile and profoundly weird. It's a testament to evolution that it works at all, given the design quirks. Much like fingerprints or snowflakes, no two penises are identical (trust me, I've seen enough in my professional capacity to have formed a mental case series), and most of what men panic about is *completely normal*. Some are smooth and unassuming, others boast a topographical map of bumps, veins and spots that could rival a Jackson Pollock painting.

Most of these quirks are unusual but not alarming, and frankly, penises deserve more appreciation for their individuality.

Spots, bumps and other curiosities

- **Pearly penile papules (PPP):** These tiny, white, dome-shaped bumps often form a neat row around the head of the penis, like nature's attempt at accessorising. Unfortunately, they're the sort of thing that send men sprinting to Dr Google late at night, only to discover they're about as dangerous as freckles. Be assured, they're benign, common and absolutely nothing to worry about. PPP is a normal anatomical variant, not a sexually transmitted infection, TI, and is more common in uncircumcised men. Think of them as the fringe on a cowboy jacket – unexpected but completely harmless.

- **Fordyce spots:** These are tiny, pale yellow or white bumps that appear on the shaft or scrotum. They are sebaceous (oil) glands, which don't open into hair follicles like regular ones, so they're more visible – and yes, they're meant to be there. They're not a disease or a sign of poor hygiene, just a reminder that even genitals need oil control.

- **Veins that could double as roadmaps:** Some penises have veins that are so prominent they look like they're auditioning for a role in an anatomy textbook. These veins are completely normal and help with blood flow during erections. Some men have thinner skin or more superficial veins, making them more visible. They might look like the London Underground map but, rest assured, they're functional and not a sign of derailment.

- **Curves, bends and banana shapes:** Not every penis stands to attention in a straight line, and a gentle curve to the left or right is perfectly normal. In fact, most penises have a degree of curvature due to how the tissues developed during puberty and the uneven tension in the fibrous tissue that surrounds the erectile chambers. It's not 'broken'; it's bespoke. Michelangelo didn't sculpt in straight lines, and neither did nature when it got to penises.

- **Uneven testicles:** While not technically part of the penis, testicles deserve an honorary mention here. One is often slightly lower than the other, which is both normal and practical as it prevents them from knocking together like clumsy conkers. You can thank the combination of anatomy and gravity for this. The left testicle is often lower due to the position of its spermatic cord. Just think of it as nature's own asymmetrical art. Just remember: they're not uneven; they're . . . ergonomic. So, the next time someone panics over an anatomical quirk, remind them: the only thing that's truly abnormal is expecting everything to look the same. After all, if you wanted symmetry and predictability, you wouldn't have signed up for the human experience . . . but then again I guess that wasn't your choice! If in doubt, blame your parents.

TIDYING THE BOTTOM GARDEN

The age-old question of whether to tame the wild underbrush: is it about hygiene, or is it just one more way society messes with our insecurities? Let's dig in (metaphorically, of course, because nobody's getting that personal here) to an issue that applies just as much — if not more — to women, who are under increasing pressure to get the full Brazilian down below.

The hygiene myth

First, let's bust the big one: trimming or shaving pubic hair doesn't make you inherently cleaner. Your body hair isn't a filthy sponge soaking up bacteria; it's there for a reason. Evolution didn't add a decorative wreath for optics alone. Pubic hair acts as a barrier, reducing friction, preventing skin irritation, and even trapping dirt and sweat to keep it from reaching sensitive areas. It's your body's natural line of defence.

Going bare downstairs can increase the risk of skin irritation, ingrown hairs and micro-abrasions that might invite infections. So, if you're wielding a razor thinking you're doing your health a favour, think again. You're probably just opening the door for some very unwelcome bacteria to RSVP to the party.

The aesthetic pressure

Now let's get philosophical: the obsession with tidying up down there isn't rooted in hygiene, but societal expectations. Somewhere along the way, modern culture decided that smoothness equates to cleanliness and, for men, masculinity. Blame it on porn, blame it on marketing campaigns for razors, or blame it on the collective fear of looking 'primitive'. The truth is, it's all about what we've been taught to find attractive.

While we're all busy hacking away at body hair to conform to an arbitrary standard, we're ignoring the fact that these norms are as ephemeral as fashion trends. What's considered 'groomed' today might be seen as weirdly clinical tomorrow. Your great-grandfather probably never thought twice about his pubes, and his love life probably didn't suffer for it, or you wouldn't be here today.

So, should you trim?

If grooming makes you feel more confident, go for it. But don't let the world convince you that your natural state is somehow inherently unclean. Your body hair, like most things in life, exists for a reason, even if that reason seems vaguely absurd at times.

At the end of the day, whether you're rocking the Amazon rainforest or a neatly trimmed lawn, what matters is that you're comfortable in your own skin. So, trim, shave or let it grow wild, but do it because you want to, not because some unwritten cultural rule told you to. Life's too short to let your grooming habits be dictated by anyone but yourself.

One thing is for certain, no matter the landscape design, there are some rules to bear in mind to stay safe when trimming or removing your pubic hair.

- Don't use the same instruments for your downstairs hedge that you use for other body parts. Just like you wouldn't share a toothbrush with your dog, you shouldn't use the same trimmers or scissors on your groin that you use for your face. Using one tool means more cross-contamination, which means there is a risk of translocating microbes (bacteria, yeast and fungi, etc.) from one place to another. To minimise spread, sterilise your tools with alcohol before and after each use and give your meat pole a good wipe down beforehand (with soap, don't get any ideas now).

- Manscaping can be an activity fraught with peril. Aside from infection, you run the risk of skin irritation, bumps, itching and rashes. To this end use trimmers on the long hairs first before switching to a razor to shave.

- Minimise the use of scented or fragrance-infused products like mineral oils, perfumes or 'flavoured' soaps or shampoos down below as it could cause irritation and affect the skin barrier.

This Is Vital Information

The anatomy of an erection

Achieving lift-off isn't rocket science when it comes to erections, although preparing for launch does rely on the coordination of complex events and the presence of basic starting materials: a strong chassis, hydraulics, adequate wiring and mission control (your brain).

The strong chassis required for erections consists of two main cylinders. Known as the corpora cavernosa (which might sound like a Harry Potter spell but isn't), these fill the shaft of the penis during the erection and engorge with blood. These elongated vessels are surrounded by a flexible tissue called the tunica albuginea (Latin for long, sleeveless white shirt – the peak of ancient Roman fashion). This tissue has the unique ability to allow your penis to expand like a balloon and simultaneously harden.

Boner science is a more intricate process than it might appear; orchestral almost. The veins that drain the blood from the penis have to traverse the walls of the shaft cylinders. At the same time, in the midst of expansion, these draining veins are pinched shut, thus trapping the blood in the erect penis. Ischiocavernosus muscles at the base of the corpora cavernosa also squeeze the cylinders and raise the pressure in the penis higher still.

Failure to launch

There might come a time when your rubber dinghy begins to nosedive. Perhaps this has already begun, perhaps you're in the thick of it, or maybe you just want to reduce the risk of it happening. Fear not, it is nothing to be embarrassed about, nor is it uncommon, despite what your locker-room chat might suggest. Around 10 per cent of men will experience it at some point in their lives.

Erectile dysfunction (ED), as the name suggests, is the inability to keep the purple-headed snake as hard and for as long as you might like. Even now the topic is spoken about in hushed tones: who would want to tell the world about their wilting flower, right?

If you have ED and it's affecting your quality of life, it's worth exploring the myriad of possible causes, medical and psychological. Addressing these might help with your erection and improve your general health in the process.

Feeding the beast

Chocolate, oysters, the aptly named horny goat weed: cultures around the world are rife with tales of certain foods that are aphrodisiacs, kick-starting your game in the bedroom. Sadly, there isn't sufficient evidence to suggest these actually work. Consuming certain foods won't have an immediate effect – what you chow down for lunch won't make you a rock star in the bedroom the same evening – but in the long term, diet *does* have a role in the strength of your erection: both directly and indirectly.

A diet rich in nitrates and antioxidants, meanwhile – vegetables, fruits, nuts, legumes and grains – can help to provide a bountiful supply of nitric oxide (which can help with blood flow) and antioxidants, which mitigate the ageing process.

None of this guarantees you the stamina of a twenty-year-old, but it can definitely stack the odds in your favour and potentially prevent a bad problem from getting worse. And if you do find yourself needing additional support, the added nitric oxide can even help with the efficacy of sexual aids like Viagra.

Talking of Viagra . . . the little blue pill has gone from failed blood pressure medication to game-changer for the sex lives of many (and improved the quality of life) but it still lives under the heavy duvet of taboo.

Erections are somehow both everywhere and nowhere in our cultural conversation. You see them euphemised in ads using grapefruit-slicing metaphors, but actual discussion of erectile dysfunction (ED) – a serious *medical* issue affecting up to 50 per cent of men over forty – is laced with shame or bravado-fuelled denial.

This Is Vital Information

Physiologically, erections require a precise neurovascular symphony. The release of nitric oxide triggers the enzyme guanylate cyclase, which boosts cyclic guanosine monophosphate (cGMP), relaxing smooth muscle and allowing blood to engorge penile tissue. Viagra (sildenafil) inhibits phosphodiesterase-5 (PDE5), the enzyme that degrades cGMP, essentially keeping the 'stay hard' signal turned on longer.

It doesn't work as an aphrodisiac and it doesn't give you a boner at the dinner table. You still need desire and arousal, so think of it more as taking your foot off the brake, rather than pressing the accelerator. However, there are men who are popping it recreationally, chasing 'super sex' without understanding that stacking Viagra with nitrates, poppers, or pre-existing heart disease can be a fast-track to cardiac arrest. Suddenly it's not so sexy.

The appropriate dose is 25–100mg taken around an hour before sexual activity and no more than once a day. And just so you know (because I can read your mind), it *won't* help performance anxiety or low libido. For that, you need a conversation rather than a chemical. More on this later, but erectile dysfunction is often a vascular red flag and the penis is simply the canary in the cardiovascular coal mine because if you find that your erections are flagging then perhaps your heart might be too.

More sleep, more boners

Broken sleep means your pituitary gland releases less testosterone. Additionally, poor sleep is a stressor so chronic sleep deprivation can increase levels of cortisol, the stress hormone, which also has an adverse effect on testosterone.

Morning glory

The morning tent pole – or the more wanky doctor name 'nocturnal penile tumescence' – is a physiological phenomenon that is an interesting marker of sexual function and general health. The reason men often wake with morning wood is probably related to the fact that REM, or rapid eye movement, sleep (the dream stage) precedes waking up.

The average human experiences several REM cycles a night and at this point of the sleep cycle testosterone levels are at their highest. In fact, men can expect around five erections a night, with each lasting up to a mighty thirty minutes.

It's also been proposed that the morning erection is influenced by the sensation of a full bladder stimulating the spinal nerves involved in producing an erection. This would also explain why erections often subside after emptying the bladder.

The brain-penis

Contrary to what most men think, the biggest sex organ is actually between your ears – yes, your brain, my friend. It processes a constant stream of information, including erotic, tactile and visual stumuli, which are turned into signals and sent down to the penis.

An erection might ensue, although anxiety, fear and negative emotions could also keep you in the floppy zone. The release of stress hormones, such as cortisol and adrenaline, can act as a circuit-breaker contributing to your flag flying at half-mast.

Besides the brain, what else can lead to erectile dysfunction?

- **Narrowed arteries:** In order to maintain an erection, the highway of blood needs to be free of traffic to ensure a smooth flow. Many conditions like high blood pressure, diabetes and heart disease cause a narrowing of the arteries, which impinges on blood flow. If you consider that the penile arteries are often around 1mm in diameter (significantly smaller than the coronary arteries supplying the heart muscle), you can see how even a slight narrowing can cause the penis to suffer. In fact, in many cases the first sign of serious heart issues might be a floppy hot dog.

This Is Vital Information

- **The electrical supply:** The circuitry also needs to be in place for the penis to receive signals from the brain and beyond. Disease or damage to the nerves from spinal cord injuries, surgery or medications can also prevent normal blood flow and short-circuit the brain–penis loop.

- **Father Time:** As testosterone levels gradually decline with age and blood flow slows, most men after the age of fifty will experience erection-related issues. From the moment we are born, we are undergoing a process of decay. When we're younger, the natural processes of regeneration and renewal ensure that we can keep a degree of balance of homeostasis against the forces of time, age and 'oxidation' (the attack from free radicals, which erode our body).

- **Ageing:** As we grow older, the natural balance begins to shift in an unfavourable direction as the smooth muscle and collagen in the walls of the blood vessels decrease in concentration and become stiffer. Even our natural production of nitric oxide, the biological rocket fuel for your wiener and proven antioxidant, begins to slow with time. To this end ensuring a rich supply of nitrates in your food (vegetables, fruits, nuts, legumes, grains) can provide some balance and a source of nitric oxide, which helps not just with the gravy maker but also general health.

- **Cholesterol:** Elevated cholesterol can damage the delicate inner lining of blood vessels, the endothecium. This leads to the accumulation of plaque and the narrowing of arteries as well as reduced blood flow to the penis.

- **Smoking:** You don't need me to spell out the downsides of smoking for general health. It's often difficult to persuade the hardiest of cigarette smokers to stop and yet when you mention it is highly poisonous to the pecker – they're all ears! Smoking wreaks the same chaos on your penis as it does to the rest of your body – the harmful free radicals and chemicals damage the blood vessels supplying the one-eyed snake. Essentially, this cuts short the supply of the essential chemical nitric oxide and gives rise to 'smoker's droop' (which I'm guessing nobody wants in their lives).

Weight loss = boner gains

Your penis is essentially a hydraulic system and, for it to perform, blood has to flow freely into the spongy tissue. When excess visceral fat (the type that wraps itself around your internal organs) takes over, it wreaks havoc on your cardiovascular system. Basically, you can't water the garden if the hose is kinked.

Obesity leads to atherosclerosis and fat can clog arteries, including the ones supplying blood to the penis. So less blood flow = weaker erections.

The endothelium (the lining of your blood vessels) also gets damaged by chronic inflammation caused by visceral fat. This means your vessels can't dilate (widen) properly, and without dilation, no amount of romance will make up for the lack of circulation.

Then there's testosterone, the hormone of vitality, libido and general swagger. Visceral fat also doesn't just sit there like a passive blob; it actively produces aromatase, an enzyme that converts testosterone into oestrogen. Excess fat can rob you of your masculinity one molecule at a time.

Lower testosterone levels, higher oestrogen levels and a libido that's reeling with nostalgia at what happened to the good old days. The cruel irony is that the same visceral fat causing this also lowers your energy levels and motivation to hit the gym, creating a vicious cycle of stagnation, self-doubt . . . and a floppy penis.

Erectile dysfunction isn't just about what's happening *down there*; it's a snapshot of your overall health. Your body, for all its miraculous engineering, isn't keen on compartmentalising its failures: when your waistline expands, your arteries clog, your hormones go haywire and your inflammatory processes go wild.

But just as bad habits can sabotage your system, good ones can repair it. Losing even a modest amount of weight (say, 5–10 per cent of your body weight) can improve blood flow, boost testosterone levels and reduce inflammation. You don't need to aim for a six-pack but give your body the tools it needs to bounce back.

More testosterone, please

Testosterone, primarily produced in the testicles, is petrol for the engine in the trousers. A hormone responsible for more than erections and men's sexual health, it affects mood, memory, bone and muscle mass, as well as hair growth on various body parts.

As a man ages, testosterone production begins to slow down. Unlike the fuel gauge in a car, however, there are no warning lights indicating that the testosterone tank is running low. While we may not be able to reverse ageing (yet) and prevent the gradual decline in testosterone, we can slow it down somewhat.

Can you tell if your testosterone is running low – the equivalent of a nearly empty warning light for your T-tank as it were? A frequently seen sign is a reduced sexual appetite or libido. You might still have normal erections but just be less interested in sex. A less obvious sign of low testosterone is fatigue, combined with poor focus and concentration. Low testosterone also makes you physically weaker with a decrease in muscle strength and endurance.

So what can cause low testosterone levels?

Modern life has a way of meddling with this delicate biological balance, insidiously stripping men of their T-levels while they're too distracted by emails and existential crises to notice. Here are four of the main culprits that lower testosterone and what you can do to reclaim your hormonal balance and give your testicles the respect they deserve.

Male health hell

1. Low vitamin D

Your testicles are, quite literally, solar-powered. Deny your body sunlight and they'll sulk like neglected houseplants. Living in a basement or hiding indoors with your gaming console isn't just bad for your social life, it's bad for your hormones too (note, this does not mean you have to expose your googlies to sunlight like you might have seen on social media).

Vitamin D is a key player in testosterone production. The sunshine hormone directly influences the Leydig cells in your testes, which are responsible for producing testosterone. When vitamin D levels are low, the Leydig cells essentially get lazy, reducing the amount of testosterone they churn out.

What to do

- Get fifteen to thirty minutes of sunlight daily (face, arms, neck and hands will do) or consider a high-quality vitamin D3 supplement if you're deficient.

- Foods like salmon, egg yolks and fortified dairy can also help, but honestly, the sun's your best bet.

2. Marijuana: the chill killer

While you're getting high to 'chill', your testosterone is in free fall, and your testicles are waving goodbye . Weed might make you feel laid-back in the short term, but hormonally, it's putting your ambition on ice.

THC (or tetrahydrocannabinol), the active ingredient in marijuana, messes with the hypothalamic–pituitary–gonadal (HPG) axis, the hormonal highway responsible for testosterone production. THC reduces the secretion of luteinising hormone (LH) from the pituitary gland, which signals to the testes to produce testosterone. Less LH means less testosterone.

THC also causes oxidative stress in testicular tissue, further impairing testosterone production. Chronic use can even lead to testicular atrophy (yes, shrinkage) and lower sperm count.

What to do

- Occasional use is unlikely to tank your T-levels, but if you're lighting up daily, it might be time to rethink. Moderation is key.

3. Alcohol: liquid courage, hormonal sabotage

That 'liquid courage' you rely on to impress people at the bar is kryptonite for your reproductive health. Drink too much, and the only thing growing is your beer belly.

Alcohol disrupts testosterone production at multiple levels. It damages the Leydig cells in the testes, inhibits the release of luteinising hormone from the pituitary gland, and increases cortisol levels. Chronic drinking also boosts aromatase activity, an enzyme that converts testosterone into oestrogen.

Excess alcohol also impairs liver function, reducing its ability to metabolise oestrogen, further tipping the balance. Heavy drinking reduces testicular function, leading to lower testosterone output over time.

What to do

- Limit yourself to one or two drinks a day or consider cutting back entirely
- Swap binge-drinking sessions for a healthier vice, like binge-watching documentaries.

4. Chronic stress: the cortisol conspiracy

Stress is like that toxic friend who overstays their welcome, eats all your food, and burns your house down for fun. And while you're agonising about deadlines or your fantasy football team, your testosterone is packing its bags and leaving the premises.

When stress becomes chronic, your adrenal glands flood your system with cortisol, the body's primary stress hormone. Cortisol and testosterone have an antagonistic relationship: when one goes up, the other goes down. Cortisol inhibits the release of gonadotropin-releasing hormone (GnRH) from the hypothalamus in the brain, disrupting the production of testosterone.

Chronic stress also reduces sleep quality, which further tanks testosterone levels since most of it is produced during deep sleep. Over time, chronic stress can even cause the testes to shrink – known as testicular atrophy – reducing their output of testosterone.

What to do

- Practise stress management techniques like mindfulness, exercise or yoga
- Prioritise seven to eight hours of quality sleep to let your body repair itself.

So, get outside, put down the joint, moderate the booze, and for the love of everything sacred, take a deep breath. Testosterone goes beyond the Hollywood trope of masculinity and 1980s bodybuilders; it's also about vitality, drive, and the refusal to let life turn you into a tired, stressed-out husk.

Testosterone treatments: the good, the bad, and the really misguided

When your testosterone levels dip into clinical deficiency, it's not just a case of feeling 'off'; it can profoundly affect your body and mind. Enter testosterone replacement therapy (TRT), a legitimate medical treatment for those with hypogonadism (low testosterone caused by disease or dysfunction).

This Is Vital Information

The legitimate testosterone treatments

For men with clinically low testosterone, doctors may prescribe TRT to restore normal levels. These treatments come in various forms:

- **Injections:** *Intramuscular (IM) testosterone injections, such as testosterone enanthate or testosterone cypionate, are administered every one to two weeks. These bypass the liver and go straight into the bloodstream, providing a stable (though spiky) increase in testosterone levels.* For those who need it, it is effective and fast acting but the downsides are that it requires regular needle pokes and can cause mood swings as levels rise and fall.

- **Gels and creams:** Topical testosterone treatments work by being absorbed through the skin into the bloodstream. The pros are that they require no needles, so are easy to use. However, there is a risk of transferring testosterone to others through skin contact (so don't hug Grandma right after applying).

- **Patches:** *Adhesive patches worn on the skin, delivering a steady dose of testosterone, are another viable alternative. Similar to gels, testosterone seeps into the bloodstream via the skin.* These provide a stable delivery of the hormone but skin irritation is common, and peeling off a patch covered in sweat is about as much fun as waxing.

- **Oral pills:** Oral testosterone undecanoate is a steroid medication that is absorbed through the lymphatic system, bypassing the liver. While there are no needles or sticky residue, these capsules are less effective at maintaining stable levels of testosterone and can irritate the digestive system.

TRT is intended for men with clinically diagnosed hypogonadism, typically characterised by low testosterone levels and confirmed by blood tests or symptoms such as fatigue, low libido, erectile dysfunction, muscle loss and mood changes. It's not for men with borderline levels who just want to 'feel better', and it's definitely not for the bro at the gym trying to outbench everyone in the free-weight section.

Natty or not

Worryingly, TRT is increasingly being used by young men for aesthetic purposes, often encouraged by gym culture and social media. The 'natty [natural] or not' debates rage; social media creating the illusion that every man is ripped, when in reality it's a tiny minority that look like a Greek statue dipped in creatine.

Men are bombarded with the idea that masculinity is measured by muscle mass, leading some to inject a shortcut instead of lifting smarter or eating better. But using testosterone when it's not medically required doesn't just mess with your hormones; it messes with your entire body.

Testosterone increases red blood cell production, thickening the blood and raising the risk of clots, strokes and heart attacks. Steroids can raise LDL ('bad') cholesterol and lower HDL ('good') cholesterol, accelerating atherosclerosis (thickening of the arteries). Taking external testosterone suppresses your body's natural testosterone production by shutting down the hypothalamic–pituitary–gonadal (HPG) axis. In non-science chat, this means your testicles can shrink, sperm production can plummet and infertility can become a real possibility.

High testosterone levels can also lead to mood swings, aggression and anxiety, commonly referred to as 'roid rage' (because of the 'ste-roids' – keep up). Testosterone abuse can also cause gynaecomastia (aka man boobs) as excess testosterone converts to oestrogen. Coming off testosterone without medical supervision can also cause depressive crashes, as your body struggles to restart its natural production, and you'll regret ever having started.

WHEN SIZE MATTERS: THE PROSTATE

Do you know what the prostate does?

If that's a no, you're not alone. Most men have no idea what function the prostate actually serves. In short, it's both a crucial organ for sexual and general health and a source of serious agony in many.

Between the base of your penis and the rectum, you have a golf-ball-sized mass of tissue – the prostate gland – which supplies the seminal fluid (semen) in which sperm survive and travel from the testicles to the outside world.

Although crucial for urinary continence and sexual prowess, the prostate can often turn rogue and either enlarge over time or become cancerous. The problem is not just the lack of knowing what this organ does, but a widespread failure in identifying symptoms linked to abnormal prostate health and then seeking advice at an appropriate time.

With age, the prostate will slowly grow. This is inevitable and, in most cases, the growth isn't cancer. However, the prostate sits in a place where it has the potential to cause problems. Wrapped around the outlet pipe of the bladder, abnormal enlargement can cause problems with urine flow, incomplete bladder emptying, back pain, an excessive urge to urinate, nocturia (needing to pee at night), blood in urine and more. All of these can insidiously impact a man's quality of life, even at mild levels of prostate enlargement, and men should consult with a doctor if they experience any of the above symptoms.

The problem is most men rarely discuss these genitourinary issues with friends, family members or partners and so fail to seek medical help when they need it. In fact, most men are unaware that they should schedule an annual prostate exam once they cross the age of fifty.

Understandably, discussing intimate matters like how often you need to wake up at night to spend some golden pennies on the porcelain throne doesn't make for the most scintillating of conversations but it is important nonetheless.

Willy Olympics

Although some may flex it, the penis isn't a muscle and it can't be directly 'trained' or exercised – there is no day of the week for 'penis day' in the gym. Despite not being a muscle itself, it is surrounded by muscles that are crucial in optimising and maintaining its function.

The bulbospongiosus and ischiocavernosus are muscles at the base of the pelvis between the scrotum and anus (the gooch, in layman's terms), which squeeze mid-orgasm to allow for propulsion of the semen during ejaculation. These muscles also help to maintain the erection via compression of the blood chambers during arousal, helping to sustain the blood within the penis so it doesn't drain out via the veins and prompt detumescence (deflation of the erection).

It therefore stands to reason that by strengthening these muscles you could slow down or prevent erectile dysfunction or at least alleviate its symptoms if you have it. So how do you do that?

Men have pelvic floors too

You've probably heard about the pelvic floor if you've spent time around a pregnant woman. But it's not just women who benefit from looking after this hammock of muscles. The muscles that help maintain erections and control ejaculation are located in the pelvic area, so training your pelvic floor could help with sexual function.

Strengthening pelvic floor muscles can also help with bladder and bowel control and it's thought that up to a third of men seeing a doctor have some degree of urinary incontinence or bladder issues, but most don't discuss it. Furthermore, up to 15 per cent of men experience faecal incontinence or bowel issues and simply brush it under the carpet (not literally, I hope). Pelvic floor issues can also occur as a result of prostate issues, pelvic surgery, constipation, chronic straining, heavy bouts of coughing, or even due to being overweight.

There are some simple strategies you can employ to strengthen your pelvic floor area that might just prevent any issues or alleviate associated symptoms.

To work the pelvic area, don't use your abs or glute muscles (you wouldn't be doing an ab crunch when trying to hold in a poop, would you?). Instead, imagine sucking in your gooch (between your scrotum and anus), or tightening the muscles around your anus. If you're struggling, try standing in front a mirror: you should see the penis retract in and up slightly at its base. Simplicity is key here. I recommend holding this position for ten seconds and then slowly releasing the hold over the next ten seconds. Repeat these steps for a set of five and have fun with your pelvis!

Doing these 'Kegel' exercises regularly over three months can benefit sexual function as much as Viagra in some cases. The other advantage of doing them is that no one will know you're doing them. You can do them while watching TV, at your desk or in meetings; I've even been known to do them during surgery!

THE HAIR APPARENT

Hair loss is the silent spectre stalking most men. It creeps in during your twenties or thirties, uninvited, one fallen strand at a time. What begins as an innocent thinning around the temples can snowball into full-blown follicular despair as the mirror reflects a crown you weren't ready to wear.

Hair loss isn't just about losing hair, it's about losing an idea of yourself. It's the slow erosion of identity, one follicle at a time, as society, mirrors and your inner critic slowly convince you that your worth is tied to the density of your scalp.

This societal obsession is an illusion. More than 50 per cent of men experience noticeable hair loss by the age of fifty, and about 25 per cent start seeing it before they reach twenty-one. Baldness isn't the exception; it could be considered the rule. And yet, we talk about it in hushed tones, as though it's a shameful secret, when in reality it's as common as morning coffee.

Studies show that hair loss can significantly affect a man's mental health, leading to lower self-esteem and confidence when the image in your head doesn't match the one in the mirror. It's a form of body dysmorphia, when you fixate on your hairline, convincing yourself everyone else is too.

I've been there. I had great hair in my early twenties: thick, wavy, the kind of hair you run your hands through when flirting. Then came the slow involuntary haircut dispensed by Father Time and biology: a thinning crown, receding temples, and the horrifying realisation that my hairline had decided to withdraw involuntarily. It affected my confidence, my self-esteem, and how I felt walking into a room. I started using the scalp treatment minoxidil 5 per cent, desperate as I was to stop the march of time. It worked, sort of, slowing the loss but not reversing it. And while I came to care less about what others thought, deep down I just wanted to feel like I did in my twenties.

Why hair loss happens

The villain in this male tragedy is testosterone and dihydrostestosterone (DHT).

Testosterone converts to DHT via the enzyme 5-alpha reductase. DHT binds to androgen receptors in the scalp's hair follicles, shrinking them over time in a process called miniaturisation. The hair grows thinner, weaker, and eventually stops growing altogether.

Other factors include your genetics. If your dad or grandfather went bald, you've got a front-row seat to your follicular fate. Stress, our old friend, is also a factor. Chronic anxiety can increase cortisol levels, which can cause a greater number of hair follicles to move from their growing phase into the resting phase before they fall out. Telogen effluvium, as it is known, can also be caused by physical injury, hormonal changes and various other factors. Deficiencies in protein, iron or zinc can also weaken hair and lifestyle factors like lack of sleep, smoking and poor scalp hygiene all conspire against your mane.

This Is Vital Information

Some men choose to embrace baldness, and there's a certain nobility in that. Shaving your head can feel like reclaiming control, leaning into inevitability instead of fighting it. But for others, the fight is worth it.

Fighting back against the follicular fates

Medical options

- **Minoxidil (5 per cent or higher):** This is a topical treatment that increases blood flow to the hair follicles and prolongs their growth phase. It works for many, but results are modest, and you need lifelong commitment. The moment you stop, the shedding will continue unimpeded.

- **Finasteride:** This is an oral medication that blocks 5-alpha reductase, reducing DHT levels. It's effective but can cause side effects like decreased libido or erectile dysfunction in some men.

- **Hair transplants:** A surgical option where hair is relocated from the back of your head to thinning areas. There are many different types, including FUE (follicular unit extraction), which transplants individual follicles, and FUT (follicular unit transplantation), where a strip of scalp is removed, divided and transplanted.

  If you do decide on any surgical options, remember always go to a certified professional. The rise of 'bargain' transplants abroad has led to horror stories involving infection and botched results.

Lifestyle interventions

- **Diet:** Hair needs protein (keratin!), biotin, and omega-3 fatty acids (e.g., eggs, fish, nuts and leafy greens).

- **Stress management:** Meditation, therapy, or just screaming into the hairless void can help (I'm joking, but humour certainly helps). Stress literally makes your hair fall out faster.

- **Sleep:** Growth hormone is released during sleep, which helps repair and regenerate hair follicles.
- **Scalp care:** Keep it clean and exfoliated to prevent build-up that could block follicles.

Avoid the snake oil

- **Rosemary oil:** The hype is real but the evidence isn't strong. While some studies suggest it may improve circulation, it's no match for minoxidil or finasteride.
- **Biotin supplements:** Unless you're deficient in vitamin B7 (which is rare), these probably won't do much for your hair loss.
- **Over-the-counter gimmicks:** If it sounds too good to be true, it probably is.

The choice is yours

The beauty of modern life is that you have options. You can embrace your shiny top: shave your head, grow a beard, and lean into the Jason Statham look. Confidence, not hair, maketh the man. Or fight it: use treatments like minoxidil or finasteride, or consider a transplant. There's nothing wrong with wanting to look like your younger self, as long as it's for *you* and not societal pressure.

Hair loss is this weirdly taboo topic, yet almost every man will face it at some point. We gossip about it, panic over it, and let it define too much of how we see ourselves. But as I've come to realise, hair is just hair. Its loss doesn't make you less of a man, less attractive, or less worthy – unless *you* let it.

If you want to fight it, fight it. If you want to embrace it, embrace it. But don't let a few strands of keratin dictate your self-worth. Confidence doesn't grow on your head; it grows in your mind. And that's something no amount of DHT can shrink.

This Is Vital Information

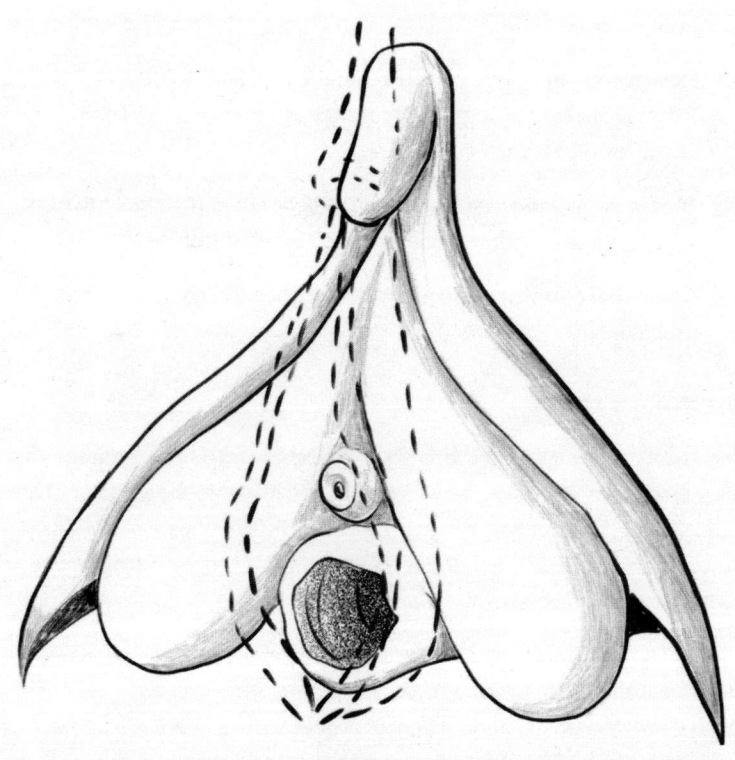

The anatomy of the clitoris

Chapter 5

PAGING DR FREUD

THE BIRDS AND THE BEES... I never really understood why that was an analogy for some horizontal bedroom ballet, but let's talk about it.

From awkwardness to embarrassment, indignation to blushing, the topic of sex arouses the full gamut of emotions and reactions. If we put aside social mores and any taboos associated with this carnal act, sex is arguably the most important thing, ever. Without it, life on Earth would not have evolved beyond simple organisms and you wouldn't be here now reading this book.

Despite being fundamental to our very existence, throughout my time in medical school I don't recall a single lecture that explored sex beyond its medical consequences such as pregnancy, STIs or embryology. Even in my postgraduate years, during rotations on urology and colorectal surgery, the focus on sexual dysfunction remained narrowly clinical, limited to pathological conditions as well as the sexual side effects of surgery that can leave a person with infertility, impotence or erectile dysfunction.

It was almost as if the medical community deleted orgasm, arousal and the nuances of procreation from the physiology curriculum; as though it were a secret shame and not an essential, everyday biological occurrence.

Thankfully, sex hasn't been entirely ignored – it's been studied in labs, documented in research, and yielded a fascinating, and often surprising, body of knowledge. For the sake of science, we owe it to the researchers, scientists and brave volunteers who battled beyond social stigma and judgement to uncover the facts. Out of respect for their efforts, we should talk about sex.

The anatomy of a snap

A&E is a confessional booth of sorts, except instead of priests you get doctors, and instead of absolution, you get antibiotics and sutures.

That's how I found myself one chilly December evening staring at a 22-year-old man with the nervous energy of someone trying to will themselves invisible. He sat hunched on the edge of the gurney, his hands fidgeting with the hem of his hoodie, trying not to make eye contact as I ran through my usual script of questions.

'What brings you in tonight?' I asked.

Slowly, in a tone that suggested he was hoping I might evaporate on the spot, he said: 'I think I broke it.'

'Broke what?' I asked, while scanning his limbs for any obvious signs of injury I may have missed.

He gestured vaguely downwards. 'You know . . . it.'

And that's how I met my first 'broken banjo string' injury; a torn frenulum of the penis, for those playing along at home. The frenulum, that delicate elastic band of tissue connecting the underside of the glans (head) of the penis to the shaft, is a marvel of human anatomy: flexible, vascular and exquisitely sensitive. It's a key player in male sexual function, aiding in the motion of the foreskin and contributing to pleasure. But like all fragile things, it has its limits.

A frenulum tear usually happens during vigorous sex, when the tissue is stretched beyond its natural capacity, a spring that's been stretched too far. In this young man's case, as he explained through fits of stammering, things had gotten 'a bit rough'. There was a sudden, sharp pain, followed by bleeding that, in his words, 'wouldn't stop'. The pathophysiology is straightforward: the frenulum, rich in blood vessels, is prone to significant bleeding when torn. Combine that with the humiliation of explaining the situation to a stranger in scrubs, and you've got a recipe for an agonising A&E visit.

As I wrote up my notes, I found myself reflecting on the dynamics of shame that had brought this man to this moment. He wasn't just embarrassed about the injury; he was embarrassed about the act itself. Sex, despite being one of the most natural and universal parts of human existence, remains shrouded in taboo.

He didn't need judgement. He needed education. He needed to know that sexual exploration, while natural, comes with risks, and that communication with a partner about comfort isn't just important, it's essential. He also needed to know that there's no shame in seeking medical help when things go sideways in the bedroom.

This wasn't my first case of sexcapade-related injuries, and it wouldn't be my last. From foreign objects to injuries from creative positions better left to Cirque du Soleil professionals, I've seen it all. And every time, the common thread is the same: shame, woven deeply into the fabric of how we think about sex and our bodies.

The genetic shuffle

Sex is the original algorithm for human connection. Long before we invented symphonies, skyscrapers or Instagram, it was sex that shaped us; biologically, culturally and existentially. Without it, there's no us.

But what began as a simple evolutionary mandate to pass on our genetic code, quickly became a cultural and psychological labyrinth. Sex is no longer just about survival; it's about expression, power and the peculiar human pursuit of meaning.

In evolutionary terms, sex is a stroke of genius (pun very much intended). It introduced genetic diversity, the secret sauce of survival (you can

This Is Vital Information

imagine a pun here, you filthy animal). Without sex, we'd still be unicellular blobs, replicating ourselves into oblivion like biological photocopiers. Thanks to recombination, the genetic cocktail-shaking that happens during reproduction, we're a species of wildly varied individuals, some of whom invent groundbreaking cancer treatment while others decide to start podcasts about UFOs. Each beautiful in their own way.

Sex, as nature intended it, is brutally pragmatic. It's a way to shuffle the genetic deck, ensuring we stay one step ahead of parasites, diseases and extinction. But humans, being the overthinkers of the animal kingdom, took sex and turned it into something else entirely: an obsession, an art form and, for many, a lifelong source of confusion.

Sex is far more than biological; it's cultural. It's the subtext of countless stories, the backbone of myths, and the not-so-subtle subject of half the paintings in the Louvre.

In many cultures, sex has been both sacred and forbidden, often within the same breath. Ancient Greek gods were basically soap opera characters with insatiable libidos, while medieval Europe turned sex into sin, selling indulgences to cleanse lustful thoughts. From Shakespeare's sonnets to Cardi B's unfiltered anthems, sex has always been the beat that drives human creativity.

For most of human history, sex and reproduction were inseparable – one led to the other, sometimes inconveniently. But then science happened and the relationship between sex and babies got, well, complicated.

The pill, condoms, IUDs and other contraceptive methods unchained sex from its reproductive consequences. Suddenly, pleasure didn't have to come with a potential side order of screaming infants. For the first time in history, people could enjoy sex purely for its psychological, emotional and physical rewards.

And if you wanted to make a baby, IVF (in vitro fertilisation) and other techniques have taken reproduction out of the bedroom and into the lab.

Paging Dr Freud

We can now create life without so much as a candlelit dinner, bypassing the act altogether. While some may lament this detachment from nature, it's hard to argue with the joy of parents who've benefited from these advances.

Despite our new-found technological prowess, we're unlikely to abandon the old-fashioned way of making babies any time soon. Sex isn't just about procreation or even pleasure, but connection. It's a way to feel alive, to assert ourselves and, sometimes, to lose ourselves entirely. Sex is one of the few human activities that exists simultaneously in the realms of biology, psychology, culture and even our salacious dreams. It's an evolutionary imperative, a societal force and a deeply personal experience. It's messy, complicated and often absurd. And yet, it's integral to who we are, both as individuals and as a species.

The first sexual revolution

In 1947, sex was less a topic of conversation and more a societal skeleton buried deep in the closet. Sure, people were having it, but talking about it was about as welcome as discussing haemorrhoids at the dinner table (I have been known to do this on more than one occasion and, now you have read chapter 1 of this book, you can too).

Then along came a zoologist named Alfred Kinsey, a man whose life's work essentially amounted to taking humanity's collective sexual repression and tossing it into the public square for everyone to gawk at. His book, *Sexual Behavior in the Human Male*, didn't just blow the lid off the subject of sex; it dismantled the lid.

Kinsey, a zoologist turned sexual sociologist, had originally spent his career studying gall wasps; small, unassuming creatures with surprisingly diverse mating habits. His transition from bugs to humans might seem odd, but it turns out we're just as varied and bizarre when it comes to reproduction. With the rigour of a scientist and the curiosity of a gossip columnist, Kinsey set out to document the previously undocumented: how, when and why humans have sex.

This Is Vital Information

The result was a tome of revelations that forever changed how society perceived sex. It turned out that everyone was a little weird in the bedroom. And by 'a little', I mean a lot.

Kinsey's data showed that the private lives of men (and later women, in his 1953 sequel) were far more varied than anyone had dared to imagine. From masturbation to extramarital affairs, from same-sex attraction to fetishes, Kinsey laid it all bare. The result was shocking, not because people were shocked by what others were doing, but because they realised they weren't alone or as singularly weird. Kinsey didn't just collect anecdotes, he turned sex into statistics. Suddenly, your quirks weren't mere pathologies, they were percentages. Are you into something unconventional? Don't worry, you're just part of the X per cent club.

After Kinsey, sex was never the same. No longer could it be dismissed as a sacred act reserved for reproduction or a sinful indulgence destined for eternal damnation. Sex was now a messy, beautiful, complicated spectrum woven into the fabric of humanity.

And yet, for all the progress, sex remains something of an enigma. It's everywhere – splashed across magazine covers, plastered on billboards, streamed into homes via every screen imaginable. But what do we really know about it? Beyond the mechanics (if you're lucky enough to even be taught that) we're taught very little about what sex does for the mind, the body or the soul.

Our scientific curiosity with coitus didn't end with Kinsey. Since then, other scientists have continued the pursuit of knowledge in the world of sex. Before we get to the scary stuff, it's worth knowing why and how sex can actually be good for your health.

Vitamin S(ex)

Science has shown that sex doesn't just feel good, it can actually do good for your body, including giving your immune system a little pep talk. Forget green juices and yoga, sex might be the ultimate wellness hack, albeit one less frequently advertised by influencers. But how, exactly, does this work? Let's peel back the sheets on the science.

Sex is a physiological symphony, activating multiple systems in the body and triggering a cocktail of hormones and chemicals that help fine-tune the immune system.

A study from Wilkes University in Pennsylvania found that people who had sex once or twice a week had 30 per cent higher levels of immunoglobulin A (IgA) compared to those who abstained. IgA is an antibody found in saliva, tears and mucus membranes. It's your body's first line of defence against pathogens entering through the mouth, nose or eyes, like a nightclub bouncer for your immune system.

Sexual activity could also promote the circulation of natural killer (NK) cells, which target and destroy virus-infected or cancerous cells. It also boosts the activity of helper T cells, which orchestrate the immune response. Think of them as the generals of your internal army, barking orders to macrophages and B cells.

Horizontal wrestling can also reduce cortisol, the stress hormone that, in high doses, suppresses immune function. Mechanistically, this happens because sex triggers the release of oxytocin (the 'cuddle hormone') and endorphins, which calm the nervous system and lower stress-induced inflammation. A happy outcome of all of this is that low levels of cortisol combined with a rush of endorphins and oxytocin induce feelings of calm, pleasure and intimacy.

The heart-pounding, blood-rushing nature of sex also improves vascular health, ensuring that immune cells travel efficiently throughout the body. Sexual intercourse and orgasm is also thought to stimulate the vagus nerve (which happens to be the longest and my favourite nerve in the body), which has a similar lowering effect on the heart rate and blood pressure.

But before you start seeing sex as the cure-all for every sniffle and cough, let's temper the enthusiasm. The immune system benefits of sex are real but subtle; it's more of a gentle nudge than a magic shield. If you're coupling up in the name of health, remember that frequency matters. The aforementioned Wilkes study found that people who had sex more than twice a week didn't experience the same IgA boost, possibly because *too much* of a good thing can stress the body, or perhaps because science wanted to teach us a lesson about moderation.

Also, let's not forget that sex is a double-edged sword for the immune system. The transmission of STIs is the unfortunate reminder that your immune system doesn't always win. Safe sex practices, such as using condoms and regular testing for STIs (sexually transmitted infections – more on that later), are essential unless you want your IgA levels duking it out with gonorrhoea.

Sex and sleep

Picture the scene: a heterosexual couple engage in some lovemaking and the guy falls asleep in the immediate aftermath. He's dared to switch off after sex – a sensitive subject in any bedroom – and his partner is rightfully annoyed. It might seem like a cliché but there is solid science behind the reason why it happens. At the point of orgasm, a veritable feast of hormones are released such as oxytocin, prolactin, endorphins and gamma-aminobutyric acid. All of these promote tiredness, a sense of relaxation and thus induce sleep.

The post-coital nap is often framed as a stereotypically male phenomenon, with plenty of jokes about men snoozing while their partners stew. But the bedroom-ballet-induced somnolence isn't the preserve of men alone. Women can also feel sleepy after sex.

Alongside the release of hormones, sex also activates the sympathetic nervous system, which is responsible for the fight-or-flight response. As a result the heart rate increases, breathing quickens, and muscles contract in rhythmic waves during orgasm. But after the climax, the parasympathetic nervous system takes over, telling the body it's time to rest and recover.

For women, the parasympathetic rebound can be especially potent, as their bodies often experience prolonged arousal and more gradual comedowns. This gradual shift into relaxation makes sleep a natural next step, which from an evolutionary perspective makes perfect sense. After successfully engaging in reproduction, or at least the pleasurable illusion of it, the body rewards you with rest.

Nature's message is clear: you've done your part; now get some rest.

UNEXPECTED ITEM IN THE BAGGING AREA

This story takes place in my second year of surgical training, in that soulless place known as the night shift.

At the witching hour of 2am, I'm called to see an elderly man in A&E with severe abdominal pain. When I start to assess him and take a history, he beckons me closer and whispers in my ear: 'I've done something terrible.'

What he told me next is one of many variations I've heard from patients based on the same 'accident'. 'I slipped in the shower and fell on the shower head,' he said, though he could easily have substituted that for shampoo bottle or loo brush handle. 'It's up my bottom.'

This man had an unexpected item in his bagging area and I was the store assistant who needed to sort out this administrative error. I've dealt with countless rectal foreign objects but this was different. His exquisite abdominal tenderness combined with the size of object that had traversed into his rectum and the mechanism of insertion led me to believe he may have perforated his colon. Not good.

I organised an urgent CT scan of his abdomen. This showed a free-floating metallic structure outside the confines of his colon associated with copious gas bubbles. It confirmed a large, vacuous hole in his intestine where there shouldn't have been one, and an unfortunate case of a sexual misadventure gone wrong. Ultimately, it ended with the gentleman in question having a portion of his colon removed and the formation of a colostomy, a stoma bag to collect his faeces.

It certainly was a bizarre sight to behold during surgery as I fished out a nine-inch rod-shaped shower head from a human being's abdominal cavity, shimmering away and still cold to touch through my double layer of latex gloves.

Why do people put things in their body crevices? The answer is always complicated, but can usually be boiled down to part curiosity and part auto-eroticism, which is a fancy term for self-induced sexual pleasure. The smorgasbord of items I've retrieved range from tiny batteries to impossibly large pint glasses fully intact. The extraction of these objects is often a rite of passage for young surgical trainees learning the ropes. They can also form the basis for unusual case reports in published medical papers and a disproportionate percentage of these cases involve males.

The fact is that foreign objects in the rectum present significant physical dangers. If we ditched the moral policing for a moment and instead provided adequate sexual education that empowered people to understand more about their own bodies, medics like me wouldn't have to listen to a string of unlikely excuses from patients about why their arseholes suffered the brunt of a supposed fall.

At its core, the shame surrounding rectal insertion isn't just about prudishness; it's about the fragile construct of masculinity. Society has long equated anal pleasure with queerness, and queerness, in too many circles, is still viewed as an affront to heteronormative ideals of masculinity.

This cultural hangover from decades of homophobia reinforces harmful stereotypes that gay men's sexuality is inherently 'deviant', which equally shames men who identify as straight. The consequence is a world where sexual exploration becomes taboo, where curiosity is punished with ridicule, and where men with perfectly treatable medical emergencies feel compelled to spin tales about errant furniture and poorly placed ornaments.

The bottom line

The rectum, biologically speaking, is an anatomical wonder. Packed with sensory neurons, it's uniquely equipped to provide pleasure and, for many, exploring this region is a natural extension of sexual curiosity. But the rectum isn't without its limits, and that's where things get dicey. Unlike other orifices, the rectum has a powerful suction force, which means objects inserted can sometimes get pulled in further than intended. Add to that the fact that the rectum curves sharply and ends in the sigmoid colon, and you have a recipe for medical emergencies.

Injuries can include:

- **Perforation:** A tear in the rectal or colonic wall can lead to life-threatening infections
- **Obstruction:** If an object gets stuck, it can block the passage of stools, leading to severe complications
- **Haemorrhoids or bleeding:** Even smaller, seemingly benign objects can cause abrasions or damage sensitive tissues.

Seek medical attention quickly – any delay could be fatal. If my patient with the hole in his colon had waited a few more hours, it's likely he would have succumbed to overwhelming abdominal sepsis (a severe infection) and not been so lucky . . . relatively speaking that is.

All things anal

I drew the short straw on a Friday afternoon, which meant I was down to cover the haemorrhoid banding clinic. Little did I know I'd be thrown a curveball.

My first patient is a young woman in her twenties suffering with haemorrhoids. I examine her bottom and notice some large, grape-like protrusions, which are clearly haemorrhoids, around the rectum wall.

Together, we go through strategies and lifestyle changes she can action to help 'reverse' her haemorrhoids.

I ask if she has any more questions and she comes at me with this zinger: 'Can I still keep having anal sex?'

It was unexpected and highlighted a rarely talked about, deeply stigmatised taboo area of sexual behaviours. As someone who devotes a great deal of time and energy to talking about guts and bums, I feel this topic deserves a few moments in the limelight.

Anal sex is, of course, commonly practised and has become increasingly popular among straight couples. Over recent decades the percentage of 16–24-year-olds in the UK engaging in heterosexual anal sex has risen from 12.5 per cent to 28.5 per cent. Despite this, there is little available information on the risks of anal sex, which might include anal sphincter injury or faecal incontinence.

To furnish you with some facts about anal sex . . . here are some findings taken from a 2016 paper on faecal incontinence and anal intercourse.

- Of the people they surveyed, roughly 37 per cent of women and 5 per cent of men had received anal intercourse in their life

- The authors found that receiving anal sex resulted in a 2.5 per cent increase in faecal incontinence risk in women and a 6.3 per cent increase in men. The authors posited this might be due to a lower resting pressure in the internal anal sphincter, which is responsible for keeping the butthole closed and keeping stools and wind firmly shut inside. Anal sex might chronically dilate and stretch the anal sphincters, causing a degree of muscle and sensory nerve damage. By extension, this can affect the sensation of sphincter control.

Another study, in 1993, also looked at the effect that anal sex had on anal function. To do so, the researchers placed balloons filled with water inside the rectums of forty men who had received anal sex and eighteen men who had not. The study found that the resting anal pressure in the men who had received anal sex was lower and mirrored the symptoms of minor faecal incontinence compared to the cohort who had had no experience of anal sex.

Beyond faecal incontinence, there is the potential for physical trauma to the anus itself and the associated microtears to the rectum. Fortunately, these tend to heal relatively quickly and are unlikely to cause major health issues beyond the increased risk of STI transmission. To minimise the risks, it is advisable to use barrier protection during anal sex.

Doctor, my penis is broken

You'll never look at the aubergine emoji the same way again. If you've followed my videos on social media, your mind might hark back to one particular offering in which I revealed a fascinating yet horrendous story of a young man with an 'aubergine deformity'. This is no culinary mishap involving eggplants. In plain terms, he had a broken penis. Yes, they can break.

While I wouldn't wish for you to allocate too much fear towards this injury, penile fractures aren't that uncommon and they deserve to be given the time of day.

Supposedly, even American basketball legend Dennis Rodman, suffered a penile fracture three times, including one occasion when he attempted a flying leap in trying to insert his meat stick into a willing partner, but ended up spraying multiple people with blood instead.

So how exactly can penises break if they don't contain bone? If you haven't been given the full primer, then here you go . . .

Humans have nothing close to resembling a bone in the penis. Even so, we know it contains two spongy tissue masses called the corpora cavernosa, enveloped by a layer of tough tissue called the tunica albuginea. As it serves to keep all the blood within it to maintain the appropriate shape of an erection, the tunica is the difference between an arousal resembling a big floppy blood-filled noodle and something with more resistance to allow for penetration.

However, during an erection the tunica, the outer envelope, becomes thin and rigid and also highly breakable.

Should the tunica rupture, which would be marked by a cracking or popping sound, this creates an opening to the corpora cavernosa, which leaks out blood. You don't need me to spell out that we're talking here about a medical emergency. At this point the swollen, purple and instantly soft penis will likely resemble an exotic vegetable. Because I care, please do not look up pictures of 'aubergine deformity' online. Or do. More education, right?

Penis breaks come down to an old nemesis of humans: physics. We're talking about a boundless force that has thwarted mankind for ever. You see, as the penis bends during a particularly savage session of horizontal bedroom wrestling, the long arc (the side opposite to the bend) becomes increasingly thinner. Now there may not be any research outlining the specifics or threshold of how many degrees of bend a human penis can take but there is a limit. And it's one not worth testing, even for scientific rigour.

The sex position with the greatest risk of penile fracture is where the partner is on top. In this position, careless thrusting can result in the penis exiting one crevice and being crushed under the weight of the bony pelvis. Sexy time, right?

A broken penis may not be life-threatening but it can be quality-of-life-threatening. Surgeons can fix the issue with stitches to close the injury in the tunica, and the earlier a person presents to hospital the better. Significant delays in seeking medical attention can increase the risk of long-term abnormal curvatures, scar tissue build-up and erectile dysfunction.

Blue balls

Blue balls is the slang term for the feelings of discomfort in the flesh marbles after a prolonged period of arousal without orgasm. There isn't much published evidence about blue balls and there has only been one case report and one questionnaire-based study in medical literature (at least at the time of writing). It is precisely this lack of evidence that has given rise to urban myths about its seriousness.

The widely accepted explanation for blue balls is an engorgement of testicular veins due to slow drainage of blood from the testicles. Typically following orgasm, the arterial supply to the testicles diminishes. This allows the veins to decompress and provide adequate drainage of blood from the crown jewels. However, a prolonged erection leads to persistent dilation of the arterial supply to the nuts. This causes compression of the venous drainage, leading to a congestion and stasis of blood in the venous supply. It is this congestion that leads to a feeling of dull pain.

The 'blue' in blue balls? Pure poetic licence. While testicles may appear slightly darker due to increased blood flow, they don't actually turn into Smurf-coloured orbs of despair.

While it is a real condition, blue balls is not a medical emergency. It's about as serious as the discomfort you feel after eating too much cheese; a minor inconvenience that resolves on its own. In fact, it typically disappears within minutes, or up to an hour at most, either through the body's natural blood-draining mechanisms or, yes, ejaculation. But – and this is important – nobody ever died of blue balls. Not one obituary has read: 'Tragically succumbed to an untreated case of unfulfilled arousal.'

While blue balls has a physiological basis, it has also been weaponised in the battlefield of sexual negotiation. Men have been known to wield it as an excuse to pressure their partners into intercourse or some form of sexual satisfaction.

The cure for blue balls? It's ridiculously simple. Here are your options:

- **Wait it out:** Blood flow will normalise on its own. It's uncomfortable, sure, but so is stepping on a piece of Lego, and you don't see people making documentaries about that.

- **Exercise:** Physical activity can redirect blood flow, reducing the sensation of heaviness. A brisk walk, some jumping jacks, or even a cold shower can do the trick.

- **Ejaculation:** Yes, the most direct cure is also the most obvious. Whether solo or partnered, releasing the pent-up tension will resolve the issue almost instantly.

That's it. No special creams, no A&E visits, no medieval poultices involving rare herbs. Just patience, movement or a bit of self-love.

THE 'MYSTERIOUS' SPECIES: WOMEN

Here are two things that have baffled and mystified scientists in the field of sexual physiology, both of which have a common bond: G-spots and female orgasms. The reasons why women and sex arrive pre-wreathed in mystery speaks volumes about the male bias in this field of enquiry. So, let's put aside centuries of patriarchy and get to the crux of the matter.

The big O

The male orgasm is pretty straightforward. Assuming he can achieve and sustain an erection, it then typically takes a few minutes of sustained stimulation to result in sexual climax and ejaculation. But what of the female orgasm?

While there are clear differences between male and female sexual experiences, it's worth stating what they have in common. In 2004 Barry Komisaruk, a psychology professor at Rutgers University conducted an *interesting* experiment. He managed to persuade some courageous couples to have sex under the scientific and radiological scrutiny of an fMRI scanner to assess their brain activity. The scans showed that during orgasm, both the men and women experienced a surge of neural activity – a kind of cognitive fireworks – which helps to explain why momentarily all other thoughts are discarded in that moment of utter ecstasy.

Differences begin to emerge, however, after orgasm. Komisaruk found that there were specific regions in the brain of men that were unresponsive to further genital stimulation immediately after orgasm. In contrast, the women's brains remained active, which aligns with the ability of many women to experience multiple orgasms. Men, on the other hand, typically need a 'refractory period' or 'break' before they can go again.

Mind the (orgasm) gap

In the middle of 2023, I had an insightful discussion with a leading sex therapist, Charlene Douglas, about the orgasm gap – a phrase coined to identify the disparity in orgasms experienced in women and men. In Britain, only three in ten heterosexual women claim to experience orgasm every time they have sex compared with three in five men. For lesbians this number jumps to two in five women, while gay men report similar numbers to heterosexuals.

So why is this? Is it anatomy, psychology, or is the patriarchy to blame?

In men, the connection between the brain and the penis is fairly direct, with sensory signals providing immediate pleasurable feedback. In contrast, the female genital area communicates with the brain through multiple nerve pathways, including those activated by clitoral and vaginal stimulation. The clitoris, often referred to as the 'seat of female sexuality', has, of course, long been misunderstood or minimised, with figures like the neurologist Sigmund Freud even proclaiming that clitoral orgasms were a sign of immaturity and were inferior to vaginal orgasms.

The complexity of sexual pleasure for women was further highlighted in another study by Dr Barry Komisaruk and Dr Beverly Whipple, which looked into how women with spinal cord injuries, where nerve pathways connecting the brain and genitals were disrupted, were still able to achieve an orgasm.

The answer lay with the vagus nerve (that favourite nerve again). Located outside the spinal cord, this vital sensory superhighway connects the brain with various organs. It can also carry information from the vagina to the brain and explained how these women could still experience sexual pleasure through vaginal or clitoral stimulation.

The G-spot

Behold the so-called holy grail of female sexual anatomy: the G-spot. This bullseye was and maybe still is prized as being the epicentre of female pleasure.

In the 1980s, the German gynaecologist Ernst Gräfenberg coined the term the G-spot – G for Gräfenberg – after describing an erogenous zone located inside the vagina on the front wall. Further research then highlighted an extensive catacomb of nerves, blood vessels and the little-known female prostate in this exact area, either side of the urethra. Later studies revealed that stimulating this area could trigger a release of fluid from the urethra – aka the pee pipe.

So what exactly is this mythical spot from an anatomical point of view? After many inconsistent studies and scant research, the prevailing theory is that it corresponds to the clitoris, which is a complex network of erectile tissue and nerves.

The small tip of the clitoris, the glans, is visible on the outside of the vulva but much of the clitoris lies beneath the surface. Its internal structure wraps around the vagina and runs alongside the urethra. (One could arguably describe the clitoris as a double penis since both are technically developed from the same embryonic tissue.) As a result, when the front wall of the vagina is stimulated it is likely the internal body of the clitoris is also stimulated.

The hypothesis was strengthened by research by Emmanuele Jannini and Odile Buisson. Using ultrasound, they demonstrated engorgement of the internal parts of the clitoris and tissue adjacent to the urethra during vaginal penetration.

All of this would suggest the path to female ejaculation should be less elusive than we might think. As a result, experts like my colleague Charlene

Douglas advise that women who find it difficult to achieve orgasm via clitoral stimulation or penetration with their partner should continue to experiment on their own until they find a way that works for them.

Sexual souvenirs

If you drive a car, you might crash. If you set foot outside, you might get struck by lightning. If you eat at a restaurant, you might get food-poisoning. And if you're canoodling, you might contract a sexually transmitted infection (STI) – which is more likely to happen than all the other scenarios.

STis are far more commonplace than society likes to admit. Unless you pledge a life of celibacy and end up in a small ashram in rural India, it's very hard to avoid them, but you can at least be aware of them and reduce your chances of catching one.

Growing up, I did not discuss relationships or sex with my parents. When watching a movie with my family, if a romantic scene came on with two characters kissing or making love, I'd squirm in my sofa seat and either make awkward conversation, fast forward the scene or briefly leave the room. Now, as a doctor, barely a day goes by when I'm not asking a patient about their sexual history or behaviour – it's all part and parcel of taking a medical history; whether they're nineteen or ninety, no one is exempt . . . nor should they be.

Perhaps by sharing some of the fascinating science around STIs, I can bring this much-avoided topic out into the open so we're all a little more comfortable talking about it.

In the name of science

Here's a lesson from history that might shed some light on why information really is power when it comes to sex and STIs.

In the year 1767 John Hunter took the yellowish penile discharge of a patient he thought had gonorrhoea and rubbed it into a wound he had created in his own tallywhacker. He (wrongly) believed that gonorrhoea and syphilis were two forms of the same disease. You could perhaps understand his confusion as at the time both diseases were known as the pox, despite having different and distinct symptoms.

Hunter persisted in his theory that the difference in symptoms of the two diseases was due to the types of tissue infected. In fact, he was so confident that he literally put his own blood sausage on the line.

Following the application of the yellow goo to his own man-piece, Hunter's notes suggested that he began to experience pain, redness and itchiness of his penis: classic and painful symptoms of gonorrhoea. To his delight, he also developed shortly afterwards painful penile sores and other symptoms of syphilis. He was pleased because he believed this proved beyond doubt that the two forms of pox were the same disease. In reality, he had developed both gonorrhoea *and* syphilis, just like the poor patient from whom he had collected his samples.

Hunter had given himself two painful venereal diseases and set back medical science for a few decades in the process. To cap it all, Hunter died in 1793 of an aortic aneurysm, probably as a result of tertiary syphilis.

Thankfully today, we know quite a bit more about STIs, so you owe it to people like John Hunter to get genned up on the subject.

What I wish more people knew about STIs

- An STI is an infection spread by sexual activity, usually by vaginal, anal or oral sex. Symptoms are wide-ranging; common signs include discharge from the vagina or penis, sores and blisters around the genitals, an itchy anus or pain while peeing.

- It's likely most people in your life have had an STI, they just don't talk about it in casual conversation. If you've never heard about

STIs outside of sex-ed classes and herpes jokes, that's because people are afraid to bring the subject up.

- You have probably dated or slept with someone who had an STI, you just didn't know because they may not have known. Most STIs are asymptomatic (without symptoms).

- People don't just get STIs because they were irresponsible or promiscuous. Some STIs, like herpes (see below), aren't only transmitted via sexual activity.

- No one deserves an STI. That's like saying somebody deserves flu.

- No sex is entirely safe sex. Condoms don't fully prevent herpes transmission, for example, and all sex poses some risk of transmitting an STI unless you know for a fact that you and your partner do not have an STI – which in reality is rarely the case.

- Thanks to the wonders of modern medicine, however, most STIs are no longer as life-altering or debilitating as they once were. In fact, if you practise safe sex and go for regular check-ups, STIs are unlikely to turn into anything particularly worrisome. For the 'classic' hits like gonorrhoea, syphilis or chlamydia, if caught early, the prognosis is good and there are very effective antibiotic treatments. In some cases, especially when asymptomatic, STIs can linger and migrate to female reproductive organs, like fallopian tubes and the pelvic area, leading to an increased risk of infertility and pain.

- You shouldn't live in fear of sex or sexual experiences but you can follow best practice: have one partner at a time, use protection, and get tested regularly. Understandably in the modern landscape of dating and hook-up culture, some people might struggle with the first bit of that advice, but the latter two can be done. Simply put, getting a regular STI screen is far easier than dealing with the longer-term consequences and possible health effects of sitting on a silent STI for weeks or longer.

This Is Vital Information

Unfriendly microscopic tenants

As a medic, I'm often the unofficial doctor for friends and family outside of work – I receive a stream of unsolicited messages, calls and sometimes even pictures or videos of skin lesions, rashes or worse (yes, exactly what you're thinking).

I distinctly remember a friend from university calling me with a panicked voice as I was heading to work one morning. 'I've just been told it's herpes. What can I do?!'

Herpes can feel like a devastating diagnosis but it is incredibly common and many people will have either mild or no symptoms initially.

So what is herpes anyway? Herpes is a viral infection caused by the herpes simplex virus (HSV), which comes in two flavours: HSV-1, usually the culprit behind cold sores on your lips, though it can also cause genital herpes; and HSV-2, the more infamous sibling, primarily responsible for genital herpes, but it's not shy about visiting the mouth either.

If you, like my friend, contract herpes you are part of a very unexclusive club. The World Health Organization (WHO) estimates that 3.7 billion people under fifty – yes, that's half the world – have the herpes STI, HSV-1, while 491 million have HSV-2. If herpes were a club, the membership numbers would put Beyoncé's fan club to shame.

Once the virus enters your body, it sets up shop in your nerve cells, retreating to its little hide-out like a bad tenant you can't evict. From there, it can reactivate whenever it pleases, causing outbreaks of painful sores or blisters.

Saying that, most people don't even know they have herpes because it often lurks silently, symptom-free. Herpes is like the overenthusiastic friend at a party: it loves to mingle. It spreads through skin-to-skin contact, whether it's kissing, oral sex or genital contact. Forget the outdated myths about catching it from toilet seats or sharing cutlery. Herpes is a lover, not a lurker. It wants intimacy, not porcelain. And no, the absence of visible sores doesn't mean it's not contagious. The virus can spread asymptomatically, slipping under the radar like a stealthy little saboteur.

While there's no cure for herpes yet, it's far from the doom-and-gloom diagnosis society makes it out to be. Managing herpes is about control, not eradication. It can be managed through antivirals like acyclovir. They don't kick herpes out of your system, but they do slam the door on its outbreaks, reducing both severity and frequency. These can be taken as needed during outbreaks or daily if outbreaks are frequent. During an outbreak, think of yourself as a very unfortunate spa guest. Use warm baths or ice packs to soothe the area and avoid clothing that could irritate your skin.

Stress, illness and poor sleep can all trigger herpes because the virus thrives when your immune system is off its game. Managing stress and staying healthy are your best defences . . . and communication; telling partners about your status and using condoms or dental dams during oral sex can help reduce transmission, though they're not foolproof as herpes likes to party beyond the barriers.

Herpes is a virus, not a verdict. It doesn't define your worth, your desirability or your capacity for love. Yes, it's inconvenient. Yes, it can be painful. But in the grand scheme of things, it's just another quirk of being human, like needing reading glasses or developing an irrational fear of clowns. And if anyone tries to shame you about it, just remember: statistically speaking, they probably have herpes too.

An unexpected gift

In 2013 the actor Michael Douglas revealed that HPV, or human papillomavirus, contracted through oral sex, was responsible for his throat cancer. The reaction was swift and predictable: late-night comedians had a field day, the tabloids churned out lurid headlines, and the public, ever eager to moralise about sex, responded with a mixture of disbelief and derision.

This Is Vital Information

But Douglas wasn't just opening up about his private life, he was sharing factual information. The science has since caught up and the evidence is clear. HPV, the sexually transmitted virus best known for causing cervical cancer, anal cancer and genital warts, can be transmitted through oral sex and is thought to be responsible for an increasing proportion of oral cancers. What's tragic isn't just the stigma Douglas faced, but the missed opportunity to have a serious conversation about sex, science and the diseases we'd rather not talk about.

HPV is not a rare, exotic infection; it's staggeringly common. According to the Centers for Disease Control and Prevention, approximately 42 per cent of adults in the US aged eighteen to fifty-nine have genital HPV, and oral HPV is estimated to affect 10 per cent of men and 3.6 per cent of women. Most of the time, it's harmless, a viral hitchhiker that our immune systems quietly clear and most people who have it do not realise and do not have any symptoms.

Of its 200-plus strains, however, there are around fourteen that are linked to cancer. Among them, HPV-16 is the ringleader, responsible for the majority of HPV-related cancers, including cervical cancer and an increasing number of oropharyngeal cancers (those affecting the back of the throat, tongue and tonsils).

Oropharyngeal cancers linked to HPV have skyrocketed in recent years, particularly in men. According to a study published in *Annals of Oncology* in 2022, HPV now causes 70 per cent of oropharyngeal cancers in the US and over 50 per cent in the UK, surpassing smoking and alcohol as the primary driver.

HPV can be spread through any skin-to-skin contact in the genital area, vaginal and anal sex, as well as oral sex. In fact, the soft tissues of the mouth and throat are susceptible to HPV infection as they lack the protective keratinised layer found on external skin, providing an easy point of entry for the virus. Oral sex can also create tiny, imperceptible abrasions in the mucosal lining, which act as gateways for HPV, and in some people the virus can integrate into the DNA of its host, triggering uncontrolled cell growth, laying the groundwork for cancer.

The good news is that since 2006 there has been a highly effective vaccine against HPV: Gardasil, and later Gardasil 9, which protects against the high-risk strains responsible for most HPV-related cancers. Yet its uptake has been shockingly low among men, despite the fact that they're now bearing the brunt of the oropharyngeal cancer surge.

The reason is partly because the vaccine was initially marketed as a 'cervical cancer vaccine', reinforcing the misconception that HPV is solely a 'women's issue'. It is rarely discussed as a risk for adults and most people associate HPV with cervical cancer in women, not throat cancer in men.

And oral sex . . . well, that's supposed to be 'safe' sex, a get-out-of-jail-free card in the roulette of intimacy. To acknowledge that it carries risks feels like a betrayal of its reputation as the harmless, fun cousin of penetrative sex. Add to that the usual anti-vaccine rhetoric, societal squeamishness about teenage sexuality, and a dose of misplaced machismo, and you've got a public health failure on your hands.

Michael Douglas's story isn't just about HPV or throat cancer but a cautionary tale about how we stigmatise sex and how it carries an undercurrent of shame in many cultures. We talk about it at low volume and then act shocked when silence breeds misunderstanding and ignorance.

What you need to know about HPV

- **HPV is normal, but serious:** Contracting HPV doesn't make you dirty or irresponsible. It makes you human. But recognising its risks, especially for oropharyngeal cancer, is crucial.

- **Vaccination is vital:** Gardasil works. If you're eligible, get vaccinated. If you have children, get them vaccinated. Protecting the next generation from HPV-related cancers should be a no-brainer.

- **Talking about it matters:** The more we normalise conversations about HPV and its risks, the less stigma it has. Michael Douglas was ahead of his time; we owe him credit for sparking a dialogue, even if it was met with laughter.

HIV

In the history of medicine, no three letters have caused as much consternation as HIV. Since the peak of the HIV pandemic in the 1980s, the damage of this disease has only been matched by the fear of HIV itself.

It was during this era, when scientists were still learning more about this novel virus, that measures were taken to isolate and quarantine those diagnosed with it, with some calls to even 'brand' or tattoo individuals with HIV as a warning to others.

Fast forward a few decades and we know that those with HIV can live a relatively normal life and even have essentially undetectable disease level, or an undetectable viral load. People with HIV who have an undetectable viral load – i.e., the amount of HIV in the blood – are not at any risk of transmitting HIV to their partners. We now also have therapy like PrEP (pre-exposure prophylaxis), which, when used correctly, is 99 per cent effective at removing the risk of catching HIV. And yet, the HIV stigma still hasn't fully disappeared.

How did we get HIV?

In the summer of 2003, my usual biology lesson was visited by a guest teacher and in her hand she had a cucumber and a condom. This biology lesson had taken an interesting turn.

After a brief demonstration of how to properly sheath a gourd, the teacher played a short, archaic sex-ed film about HIV and STIs from the early nineties. Job done, we quickly resumed our usual biology class.

Paging Dr Freud

In the lunch break after this lesson, schoolboy banter took over as we joked about how big or small everyone's model cucumber was and chided each other as teenagers are wont to do. When it came to the topic of HIV, which was mentioned in the short film, one boy curiously posed the question: 'Where did it come from?'

Another boy, with supreme confidence, blurted out: 'Some humans having sex with monkeys!' Shrieks of laughter echoed through the science building corridors as the group of boys sped off to lunch. I didn't know much about HIV at this stage but this childish remark provoked my curiosity. Where did it come from?

This myth is quite a common and pervasive one. However, science has concluded that HIV in the human population likely originated around 1921 from a bush hunter in central Africa, who was exposed to the contaminated blood from an ape that was hunted and killed for food. The myth of HIV coming from sexual contact with apes is sadly another example of the long history of racist rhetoric in medicine.

The virus then disseminated across Africa. In this specific case the spread was slow as it requires the exchange of bodily fluids typically through sexual transmission, blood transfusion and sharing needles. From Africa it was exported to Haiti in the 1960s, before making a quick journey to the US at the beginning of the seventies and its spread accelerated via transmission in the gay male community.

What to do if you think you have been exposed to HIV

I came across a video, on social media of course, in which a young woman with HIV posted a question to her audience: 'Should I tell the nail salon that I have HIV?' The comment section was a dumpster fire of prejudice, ignorance and peak fear-mongering, with many people worried that they too could contract HIV if they used the same equipment.

> ### *Can you get HIV from a nail salon?*
>
> While technically being exposed to another person's blood can be a conduit to transmitting HIV, there are no documented cases of nail salons being a hotspot for HIV transmission or nail trimming as a high-risk exposure activity.
>
> Fingernails themselves don't have blood vessels, so for this to be even the remotest possibility, a person with the virus would need to cut themselves and bleed on to equipment, which would then be used by another person who also happens to have a wound. Even this scenario, unlikely in itself, would be unlikely to yield a transmission. HIV, like other STIs, has very poor survivability outside of the human body.
>
> That said, one would hope most nail salons have strict hygiene practices and clean their equipment before using it on new customers as there is more risk of other contact-related medical issues like ringworm – but these don't provoke the same level of public anxiety.

PEP

A few years back I was conducting an emergency operation with a junior colleague. The patient we were treating revealed he was HIV positive and hadn't been consistent with his antiviral treatment, so we took some extra precautions during the operation. Despite this, my junior colleague ended up stabbing himself with his own needle while stitching – more common than I'd care to admit for us surgeons – and drew blood.

As recently as twenty years ago, this experience would have caused panic across the ward, but fortunately we now have a clear procedure to follow in these instances. My colleague was prescribed PEP and returned to work not long after.

PEP is a medical Hail Mary for when safe-sex precautions fail. Think of PEP as the fire extinguisher of sexual health – something you hope you'll

Paging Dr Freud

never need to use, but if you do, you'll be very glad it exists. It's not a magic undo button for risky encounters, but it's about as close as science gets to hitting 'Control + Z' on potential HIV exposure.

PEP stands for post-exposure prophylaxis. It's a twenty-eight-day course of antiretroviral medication designed to stop HIV from establishing a foothold in your body after a potential exposure. But don't mistake it for a casual back-up plan; PEP is serious business, requiring commitment.

HIV works by hijacking your immune cells (specifically CD4 T-cells) and turning them into virus factories. PEP's job is to slam the brakes on this process. The medication interferes with HIV's replication machinery, keeping it from spreading and embedding itself in your system. Essentially, PEP shuts down the party before it even gets started.

But timing is everything. You need to start PEP within seventy-two hours of exposure, and the sooner the better. Think of it like trying to stop a train; once it's picked up speed, it's a lot harder to slow down.

PEP isn't over-the-counter medication. You'll need to see a doctor, go to an A&E department, or visit a sexual health clinic. They'll assess your risk and, if appropriate, prescribe PEP. It's usually prescribed in cases of high-risk exposure, such as unprotected sex (anal or vaginal) with someone who's HIV-positive or whose status you don't know, and needlestick injuries (a common scenario for healthcare workers).

The sooner you start, the better your chances of stopping the virus in its tracks and PEP usually involves a combination of two or three antiretroviral drugs taken once or twice daily. Missed doses can reduce effectiveness and PEP can come with side effects like nausea, fatigue or headaches. It's not a picnic, but it beats the alternative. After finishing PEP, you'll need follow-up HIV testing at four to six weeks, three months and possibly six months post-exposure to confirm that the virus hasn't snuck through.

If you're in a scenario where you're worried but don't qualify for PEP, consider PrEP (pre-exposure prophylaxis), which works by stopping HIV getting into your body in the first place. It's like building a firewall instead of waiting to put out a fire.

PEP is not a Plan B for HIV prevention. It's an emergency measure, not something you should rely on repeatedly. PEP does not protect against other STIs or pregnancy. So if you're worried about gonorrhoea, chlamydia, or an unplanned baby, PEP isn't going to help you there. PEP also isn't 100 per cent guaranteed. If you start late, skip doses, or have a particularly high-risk exposure, there's still a chance of infection.

Syphilis

When we think about STIs that ran rampant and turned into full-blown epidemics, HIV/Aids usually tops that list. But if you look through the annals of history, you'll find another epidemic that caused widespread moral panic and stoked xenophobia. In fact, this particular epidemic lasted centuries and caused untold physical suffering, and the fear of it across the globe was even exploited as a geopolitical weapon.

One of the first recorded documentations of the disease in Europe was around 1495 in Naples, shortly after the French had invaded the shores of Italy – the Italians quickly named it *il male francese* and in turn the French called it *la maladie napolitaine*. And so began centuries of passing the buck while the disease slowly spread across the world. Note: this isn't the first time that the finger of blame has been pointed at another country for a disease: think Donald Trump calling Covid-19 the 'Chinese virus', while the 1918 influenza epidemic was known unfairly as the 'Spanish Flu'.

Syphilis ran rampant for a long time and the roll call of those affected probably includes many people's 'dead or alive dinner party guests': Van Gogh, Nietzsche, Gauguin, Beethoven, Dostoevsky and likely countless more.

Thankfully for the French and Italians, we've moved past the name-calling stage of this rotten disease, though it still affects something in the region of 0.5 per cent of adults globally (in 2022 that equated to around 8 million new infections across the world). Since the advent of penicillin in the early twentieth century, syphilis has become a treatable disease. Despite this, it still leads to hundreds of thousands of – preventable – deaths every year.

Pain and pleasure

There is something about pain when mixed with sex that creates a heady cocktail of taboo. Sex and pain are like forbidden lovers and have fuelled the imaginations of script writers and authors throughout history, from the Marquis de Sade in eighteenth-century France to E.L. James's *Fifty Shades of Grey*.

Pain and pleasure. Two sensations that, at first glance, seem about as compatible as a nun at a heavy metal concert. Yet, for some, pain during sex isn't just tolerable, it's enjoyable, even desirable. This isn't a glitch in the matrix of human sensation; it's a feature of the remarkably complex and occasionally perverse thing we call the human brain. So, why does pain sometimes feel good, especially in the bedroom?

The secret to this mystery lies in the overlapping circuitry of pain and pleasure in the brain. You see, pain and pleasure aren't processed in neatly separated zones like cubicles in an office. They're entangled, sharing some of the same neural pathways.

The brain interprets pain differently depending on the context. Stubbing your toe on the leg of a coffee table . . . well, that's just plain annoying. A light slap during consensual sex . . . that's a different story. Pain isn't just a physical experience; it's deeply psychological. In the context of consensual sex, pain takes on a whole new meaning. It's no longer a threat but a choice. And that choice can be empowering, arousing and liberating.

When you experience pain, your body responds by releasing endorphins, those lovely little chemicals that act as natural painkillers. Endorphins don't just dull pain, they also stimulate the brain's reward system, creating a sense of euphoria. Essentially, your brain tricks you into feeling a cocktail of emotions – both 'Wow, that hurt', but also 'Wow, I feel great!'

This Is Vital Information

Pain and pleasure both activate the brain's nucleus accumbens, a key part of the reward system. This overlap explains why, under certain circumstances, the two sensations can blur together, creating an intoxicating cocktail of stimulation.

Add a dash of dopamine, the brain's feel-good neurotransmitter, into the mix and you've got the perfect recipe for arousal. The anticipation of pain or the thrill of doing something taboo can trigger a dopamine surge, heightening sexual pleasure.

In consensual BDSM (bondage and discipline, dominance and submission, sadism and masochism), for example, trust between partners plays a huge role. The knowledge that pain is being inflicted in a safe, controlled environment can transform it from something harmful into something thrilling. The brain's prefrontal cortex, which governs decision-making and emotional regulation, gives the green light.

Functional MRI scans show that the brain regions activated during pleasurable sexual experiences overlap significantly with those activated during certain types of pain. This overlap includes the insula and the anterior cingulate cortex, both of which are involved in processing emotions and bodily sensations.

Of course, this isn't to say that pain during sex is always good. Pain caused by a medical condition is an entirely different matter. If something hurts and you didn't sign up for it, that's your body's way of raising the alarm.

Unwelcome pain

Unless it's intended, the simple act of sex should not be painful. There is nothing in the physiology or biology of coitus that should incite pain unless there is an issue with the hardware. In simple terms, if something doesn't feel right, then something is probably going wrong.

Dyspareunia is the medical term for painful sex, or discomfort that occurs before, during or after intercourse. Non-penetrative sex, i.e., stimulation of the genitalia or perineum, the area between the anus and vagina, can also trigger pain.

A wide range of conditions can cause pain during sexual contact, from physical injuries and skin disorders to STIs, hormonal changes, such as those experienced during menopause, and pelvic floor dysfunction. In some cases, painful sex can be an indication of an underlying gynaecological condition such as endometriosis or ovarian cysts.

Pain during sex is surprisingly common and more women are affected than men, with estimates suggesting that 75 per cent of women experience pain during sex at some point in their lives, either as a one-time occurrence or as a more long-term issue. In some cases the pain is caused by vaginismus, when the muscles surrounding the vagina involuntarily contract in response to penetration. This can be triggered by psychological factors, such as fear or anxiety, or by physical conditions like endometriosis or an STI.

If men experience pain during sex it can be caused by a host of conditions, from a simple skin allergy or an issue with the foreskin (such as dryness, tightness or inflammation) to an STI or prostatitis (inflammation of the prostate gland), which can cause pain during or after ejaculation.

The unfortunate reality is that there's still a deep-rooted belief – fuelled by popular culture, movies and especially porn – that pain equals 'good' sex and that if a woman appears to be in pain, it means the man is 'doing it right'. This idea is dangerously misleading, especially for the countless young teens absorbing these messages as a form of virtual, and very flawed, sex education.

Beyond the stigma itself, the physical pain alone can cause many sufferers to avoid relationships and sexual intimacy altogether. Just as we've seen a slow and steady thawing of mental health stigma in recent years, it's time for sexual health stigma to undergo the same shift.

This Is Vital Information

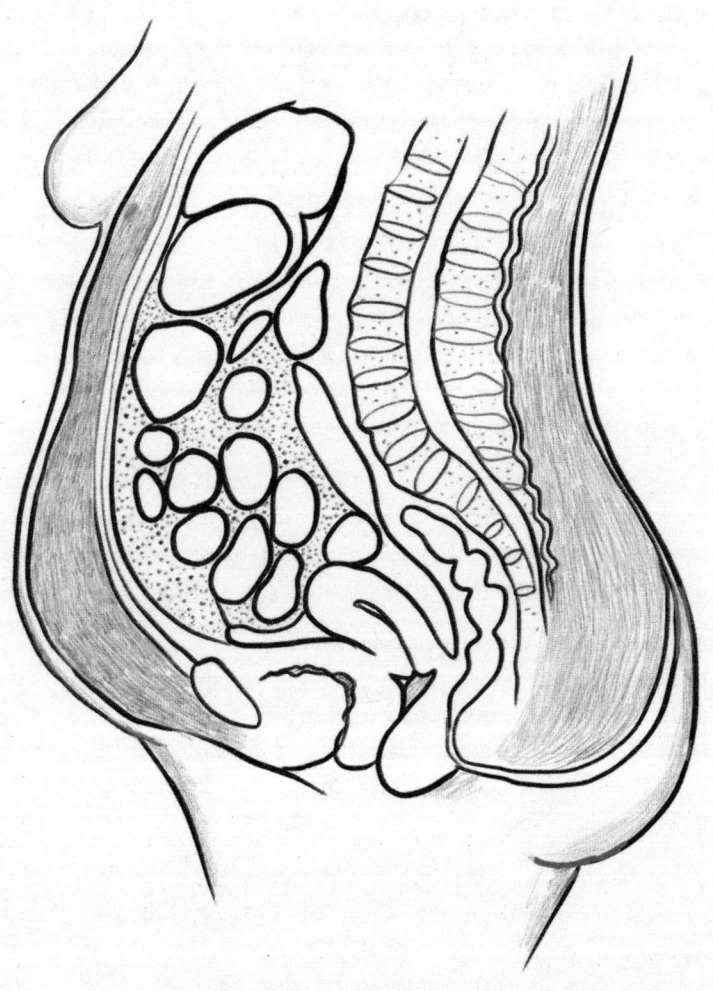

The layers of fat in the stomach

Chapter 6

WEIGHT LOSS WEIRDNESS

IN MY SECOND year of medical school, one thing I particularly looked forward to after the summer break was going back to the anatomy lab. I don't know if that reveals some dark underbelly to my psyche but my spirits were high. Despite coming to the end of a wonderful eight-week hiatus from essays and revision, I would be dissecting and exploring the wonders of human innards.

New year, new cadaver. The body that lay before me was of a large man in his fifties. Once I began the dissection, the first thing that revealed itself to me was a glistening, translucent, one-inch carpet of fat across the abdomen. It glimmered with the radiance of mildly aged cheese and made a squelching sound as the scalpel carved through it to get to the deeper layers.

Fat is often viewed as a structure that lies dormant beneath the skin. It's the body's biological doormat before you get to the good stuff inside. Beyond this outer layer, as I explored the abdominal cavity, I found more fat cuddled around various organs. There were greasy blankets of fat draped over the intestines, dollops of fat dangling from the edges of the colon like Christmas baubles and in practically every corner of the body.

I pondered the life this man had lived. I wondered how the generous stores of body fat had influenced his life. Did it put strain on his internal organs, his musculoskeletal system, or even block his arteries? More than likely he suffered the pervasive stigma of being overweight, his condition affecting probably every aspect of his life. And he is far from alone. There are millions more like him and yet many medical professionals have an extremely limited understanding of body weight, obesity, diet and nutrition. Let's first take a look at what we mean by fat and its many different guises.

THE DIFFERENT FACES OF FAT

Whether it's on social media, in magazines or on TV shows about health and fitness, you'll often be told how to burn, blast or blitz fat. While fat often gets a bad rap, dismissed as a villainous substance and unsightly impediment, the puzzling nature of fat continues to defy standard assumptions. I mean fat is just fat, right?

Science is only just beginning to understand the many different nuances of body fat. Also known as adipose tissue and adipocytes, our fat cells carry out myriad tasks key to the proper functioning of your biological machine. These roles range from storing energy and providing insulation to facilitating immune responses and even influencing our metabolisms. And yet they can turn rogue and rebel if overworked.

Body fat is a remarkable beast. It has an unparalleled ability to stretch itself and balloon well beyond its original size and then shrink down again with remarkable flexibility. Under normal circumstances adipocytes store excess nutrients in the form of lipids to prevent them from collecting in other tissues, where they can cause inflammation and anarchy. As these biological microscopic sponges absorb fat, they swell up and when they deflate they can release it.

The fat cells also release adipokines, hormones that can affect metabolism, regulate satiety signals (the feeling you've had enough to eat) and play a role in inflammation. These fat storehouses are an excellent source of on-demand energy built up in times of feast and ready to be used if famine strikes.

However, when they become overloaded with nutrients and grow too large, they can be starved of oxygen and die. The death of a fat cell sets off a chain reaction of harmful effects that ultimately contributes to high blood pressure, high blood glucose and metabolic dysfunction. This process can happen in people with normal body weight too, but in obese individuals there is a greater chance of the fat malfunctioning since the existing adipocytes are often larger.

There are three types of body fat: white, brown and beige. White fat is the most common type and is further broken down into visceral fat (which lies deeper and surrounds organs) and subcutaneous fat (the kind you can pinch when you grab a handful of belly roll). The white fat stores energy and plays an important role in hormone production and function.

Brown fat produces heat to insulate you and is often deposited in locations around the spine and collarbone. White fat cells can turn into beige cells when the temperature drops and start to behave as brown fat. They can also revert back to white fat when temperatures climb again.

Visceral feelings

If we were to label one type of fat as the villain, it would be visceral fat. This is the stuff that lurks deep inside the body recesses and makes up around 10 per cent of your body fat. High amounts of visceral fat have been linked to a higher risk of metabolic conditions including diabetes, cardiovascular disease and certain types of cancer.

Visceral fat gets a bad rap because it's extremely biologically active. This means it produces hormones and other chemicals that can affect other tissues and substances like cytokines and proteins that can constrict blood vessels and raise blood pressure.

Genetics and age influence how much visceral fat you store in your body but there are plenty of ways to keep it under control.

Studies show that both exercise and calorie restriction can reduce visceral fat and contribute to weight loss. Interestingly, though, it is only exercise that shows a dose–response relationship with visceral fat. That's to say, increasing your amount of exercise results in a greater degree of visceral fat loss. Calorie restriction, meanwhile, is *not* dose-dependent, meaning that fewer calories does not equate to greater visceral fat loss after a point.

While both interventions achieve fat loss via the mechanism of creating an energy deficit, there seems to be some key physiological differences between exercise and calorie-cutting. Importantly, when reducing calorie intake, some of the body weight loss includes a loss of muscle mass (a very metabolically active tissue), which results in a lower metabolic rate. As a result, you need an even greater reduction in calorie intake for continued weight loss, the cycle continuing with diminishing gains.

In contrast, fat loss achieved through exercise is more likely to preserve muscle tissue. Even without weight loss or calorie restriction, a study has shown that exercise can reduce visceral fat by 6.1 per cent while a lowered calorie intake without exercise showed no significant change.

Cardiovascular exercise

Anything that increases your heart rate and effort for prolonged periods of time (get your mind out of the gutter) will help to target visceral fat.

My top suggestions for a fat-busting fitness regime would be a moderate-to high-intensity cardio workout, up to sixty minutes max, three times a week. To work out what 'moderate' means, you should figure out your maximum heart rate (in crude terms, this should be 220 minus your age) and then calculate 75 per cent of that figure. Your final number should roughly equate to your heart rate during a moderate-intensity workout.

Weight loss weirdness

What to eat to reduce fat

From a nutrition perspective, studies like the DiRECT randomised controlled trial and its four-year follow-up suggest that a Mediterranean diet, rich in unsaturated fats and fibre, can improve cardiometabolic health and reduce visceral fat even without significant changes in body weight.

When it comes to nutrition, fibre is the powerhouse – not only does it make you feel full but it provides other health benefits, including reducing visceral fat. Soluble or fermentable fibres absorb water to form a gel-like consistency, which slows down the transit of food in the GI tract, helping a person feel fuller for longer while also reducing the absorption of calories from other food.

There's one other incredible role fibre can play in facilitating weight loss. You've no doubt heard of weight-loss treatments like Wegovy or Ozempic. These contain the active ingredient semaglutide, which regulates appetite, reduces hunger pangs and results in weight loss.

Semaglutide is a mimic of a hormone your body naturally produces when you eat food, known as GLP-1. The good news is you can make more of this hormone. It won't offer the same potency as weight-loss medication but it could certainly improve satiety and reduce cravings.

Ultra-fibre

To understand how fibre can help with satisfaction, let's take a look at what happens when you don't consume enough of the stuff. You wake up in the morning feeling ravenous and shovel down a couple of pieces of toasted white bread with butter. The crushed and pulped food makes its way into the small intestine, where the carbohydrates and other nutrients trigger a waterfall of activity through your bloodstream and brain.

When food enters the intestine, the cells lining it signal the release of multiple hormones, some of which help regulate the feeling of fullness.

This Is Vital Information

This includes our friend GLP-1, which stimulates the release of insulin and causes a slowing down of food transit, so you don't burn through all the fuel in one go. GLP-1 also has a role in manipulating your brain and the motherboard circuitry. This is mediated by the 'mini brain' in the gut, which sends signals to the brain to dial down those hunger pangs.

The only difference between our natural GLP-1 and the synthetic stuff found in weight-loss medication is that the hormone in our bodies degrades rapidly, sometimes within a couple of minutes. A couple of hours after your breakfast with limited fibre, your GLP-1 levels take a nosedive and when lunchtime appears . . . your hunger strikes again.

In contrast, the active ingredient in weight-loss drugs – the semaglutide – sticks around for days and this stability allows the drug to act on the brain for longer to reduce those cravings and appetite.

OK, so now imagine you've replaced the toasted white bread with multigrain bread or some rye bread – both higher in fibre to the tune of 10g overall. This beefy portion of fibre results in the release of more GLP-1 over a few hours after breakfast as the satiety hormones last longer after a meal with fibre. The reason for this is your body can't fully break down fibre so it travels through the small intestine relatively unperturbed and it takes around four to ten hours after a meal for it to reach the swamps of your colon. Here it encounters bacteria that can digest fibre, which then produces compounds that trigger the release of hormones like peptide YY (PYY) and more GLP-1 hours after a meal. As a result, your cravings in between meals are reduced and you can go longer without a trip to the kitchen.

The types of fibre that are particularly effective at suppressing appetite are 'fermentable' fibres, those that can be broken down and fermented by beneficial bacteria in the colon. These can be found in foods like beans, oats, lentils, greenish bananas, mangos, pears, apples, root vegetables and onions.

Weight loss weirdness

'Natural Ozempic'

While fibre can stimulate your body's natural GLP-1 production and can have a huge role to play in weight loss, don't believe claims you may have seen on social media that foods or natural weight-loss remedies can mimic the power of pharmaceutical medications.

It's like comparing a sparkler to a firework finale. Foods create a quick flicker of GLP-1, lasting minutes to a few hours. Weight-loss medications like Ozempic consist of pharmaceutical-grade, lab-engineered molecules that bind to GLP-1 receptors with laser-like precision and are designed to stay active in your system for up to a week. Sadly, no food, herb or ancient root dug from the sacred soils of Instagram wellness pages can replicate this.

Beyond fibre, however, there are other types of foods that can help to reduce appetite at least for a short while.

- **Protein:** Protein triggers the release of PYY and GLP-1, and also reduces the hunger hormone ghrelin. It makes you feel fuller for longer, but again this is a meal-to-meal effect, not a week-long appetite freeze. Typical foods: lean meats, eggs, Greek yoghurt, tofu, legumes, etc.

- **Fats:** Dietary fats stimulate the release of cholecystokinin (CCK), which slows down gastric emptying, making you feel full. The effect: prolongs satiety, but don't overdo it as calories still count. Healthy fats to eat include avocados, nuts, olive oil, fatty fish, etc.

- **The 'gut–brain axis' effect:** Your gut is lined with enteroendocrine cells that communicate with your brain. Fermented foods *may* support a healthy gut, indirectly influencing appetite regulation. While research is limited, eating fermented foods may result in subtle mood and appetite shifts, but no microbial kombucha is out there mimicking Ozempic. Foods include kimchi, sauerkraut, kefir, yoghurt, etc.

What you can do to regulate appetite:

- **Eat more soluble fibre:** Aim for 25–30g/day
- **Prioritise protein:** 20–30g per meal to optimise satiety signals
- **Include healthy fats:** Add moderate amounts to slow digestion and support hormone release
- **Eat at a set time:** Regular meals help regulate satiety hormones
- **Prioritise sleep and reduce stress:** Poor sleep and chronic stress mess with hunger hormones like ghrelin and cortisol.

If someone's trying to sell you 'natural Ozempic' in a bottle, bar or berry, just know you're buying into a fantasy. Ozempic is a drug. Broccoli is broccoli. No amount of chia seeds will replace pharmacology. Unless you can convince your pancreas to start moonlighting as a pharmaceutical factory. In which case call me. We'll patent it.

The sleep diet

Diet and nutrition are rightly seen as cornerstones of improving health but it's easy to side-step the gargantuan role sleep plays in multiple body systems, particularly metabolic health. Chronic sleep deprivation is very strongly associated with increased visceral fat storage.

Not getting enough sleep can significantly disrupt your hunger signals and your body produces less leptin, the hormone that makes you feel full, and more ghrelin, which triggers hunger. This can affect your food choices and behaviour, and often lead to overeating. Sleep deprivation also comes with a rise in cortisol levels, which encourages the storage of visceral fat around the abdomen.

Weight loss weirdness

The world of weight-loss drugs

Ozempic and similar weight-loss drugs might be hailed as a miracle and, don't get me wrong, they are groundbreaking, but they do perpetuate the cultural obsession with extreme weight loss, which is often targeted at women. Doctors and pharmaceutical companies have been involved in the enterprise of weight loss for centuries, some of which has had deadly consequences.

Armed conflict has always been a driver of medical innovation. During the First World War, it was noted that workers who came into contact with the explosive dinitrophenol lost significant amounts of weight. Within a few years, it was introduced as a weight-loss drug. However, shortly after it was licensed for use, reports of serious side effects – including blindness, nerve damage and even death – began to surface and it was banned in 1938.

In the 1940s, the amphetamine Benzedrine, which was originally used as a stimulant to keep soldiers alert on the battlefield during the Second World War, was later repurposed as a weight-loss pill, with housewives the primary market. Taking it carried serious risk, leading to cardiovascular illness, addiction and mental health issues, which in turn led to it being removed from the market in the 1970s.

A whole barrage of weight-loss treatments followed, from laxatives to thyroid medications, diuretics and more amphetamines. Then came the deadly fen-phen disaster in 1985. Fenfluramine-phentermine was shown to induce huge weight loss but along the way it was revealed to also cause fatal heart valve abnormalities.

Ozempic and other GLP-1 agonists (substances that raise the level of the GLP-1 hormone) are game-changers in that they are, as far as we know based on the studies we have to date, relatively safe and enable controlled weight loss in many patients who would otherwise have had to undergo major intestinal surgery in the form of gastric bypasses and other forms of weight-loss surgery with significant complication risks.

While most people are looking to lose fat there have been others who have gone to great lengths to procure it, sometimes via nefarious means.

The sordid history of making money from fat

It happened after a school day in the year 2000. I got home and watched one of the greatest films ever (in my opinion) on the television: *Fight Club*. One iconic scene that will be permanently burned into my hippocampal memory is the moment when the two main characters harvest human fat from the disposal bins of a liposuction clinic to create soap. There and then, I decided that I wanted to get into something just as visceral for a living. I didn't fancy my chances as an underground fighter, and so I studied medicine.

More than two decades later, I entered a rabbit hole in which I discovered that the procurement of fat is nothing new. It has been an important ingredient in pharmacopoeia for hundreds of years.

The renowned sixteenth-century physician and anatomist Andreas Vesalius instructed fellow anatomists to collect the fat from the corpses used for anatomical dissections so that it could 'obliterate scars and foster the growth of nerves and tendons'. Human fat, during this time, was thought to be a wound-healing accelerant. In fact, in 1601, during the bloody Siege of Ostend, vulture-like Dutch surgeons would harvest fat from the dead corpses on the battlefield to tend to their own soldiers' battle wounds.

Slicing up a corpse to remove fat is one thing, but how do you estimate how much body fat a person has if they are very much alive?

Health at every size and the obesity paradox

Can you be overweight and healthy? It's a question that surprisingly doesn't have a straightforward answer. Most researchers and scientists will agree that for the 'average' person a body weight of 150kg isn't healthy. (It's worth repeating here, though, that many healthy people don't fall within the category of 'average'. One hundred and fifty kilos may well be perfectly fine for a professional body builder more than 6 feet tall, for example!) Significant adiposity (the amount of fat in the body) for the average person can result in the disruption of the function of the fat cells we discussed earlier, leading to insulin resistance, elevated blood glucose and the risk of chronic metabolic disease.

The question of whether a few extra kilos poses the same risk as excessive weight is controversial, with many views and hypotheses. In fact, researchers have reached differing conclusions on real-life epidemiological studies. Without getting into the war of research words that's plagued the metabolic literature, one thing is abundantly clear: a huge diaspora of people are wrongly labelled as overweight due to inappropriate BMI usage.

The big issue with BMI

Today, the medical profession uses BMI (body mass index), a calculation that estimates body fat and whether someone is a healthy weight for their height. It is calculated by dividing weight in kilograms by height in metres squared. Measurements are then categorised into ranges: underweight (BMI less than 18.5), healthy weight (BMI between 18.5 and 24.9), overweight (BMI between 25 and 29.9), and obese (BMI 30 or higher).

BMI is often used by the medical profession to assess a person's risk for health problems and can have life-changing consequences. If it's over a certain number, for example, it might delay certain types of surgery or treatments. The stigma attached to BMI extends deep into the medical profession too, with many patients receiving unfair judgement based on it. It's no surprise that higher BMIs are linked with poor self-esteem as well as higher rates of depression and anxiety. And yet as a health metric BMI is deeply flawed.

Given we place so much weight — emotionally and clinically — on this singular metric, you'd think it was because it was based on rigorous science and evidence. But it wasn't created by a doctor and was never intended to evaluate individual health.

In the nineteenth century, Belgian mathematician Adolphe Quetelet introduced BMI to the world. In essence, it was a quick formula to measure obesity in the general population to assist in resource allocation. Used for statistics, the metric can work if you're using large sample sizes and mean values, but it was never intended to assess individuals, predict disease or whether you should skip dessert.

It's also worth noting that Quetelet based his formula on measurements from northern European Caucasian men. It doesn't account for women, people of colour or the vast diversity of body types.

Additionally, BMI takes no account of muscle mass, fat distribution or age. We know that, on average, females have less muscle mass and more fat than the average male. We also know that the proportions of muscle mass will shift with increasing age, and that genetics play a huge role in determining fat percentage. Ultimately, BMI lacks accuracy and misses many important factors that determine your disease risk and should not be the only marker of health used before deciding on treatment plans.

And yet, here we are, still treating BMI like gospel truth. If you're looking for a better predictor of health and fitness, the good news is that alternatives exist.

- **Waist-to-hip ratio (WHR)**
    - WHR measures fat distribution, which matters because visceral fat (around your organs) is a greater health risk than subcutaneous fat (under the skin).
    - **How to measure:** Divide the circumference of your waist by that of your hips. A ratio of >0.85 for women or >0.90 for men suggests higher risk of poor health.
- **Body fat percentage**
    - It distinguishes between fat and lean mass (muscle, bone, water).

- **How to measure:** You can use calipers, bioelectrical impedance scales, or more high-tech options like DEXA scans (dual-energy X-ray absorptiometry scans, which measure bone mineral density) – if you've got the cash.

What I need you to know:

- **Stop obsessing over a single number:** Health is a mosaic, not a painting-by-numbers picture. BMI is one crude tile in a much larger masterpiece.

- **Focus on habits:** Eat more plants, move more often, sleep better, and manage stress. These things matter far more than your BMI ever will.

- **Listen to your body:** If you feel strong, energetic and pain-free, you're likely doing something right.

- **Consult professionals:** A doctor or dietician can guide you towards better assessments tailored to your unique needs.

The problem with BMI is not just inaccuracy, but reductionism. It takes a complex, dynamic human being and boils them down to a single, soulless number. But health isn't a number. It's a feeling, a lifestyle, and a relationship with your body that changes over time.

So stop letting BMI bully you. Measure what matters, embrace what works, and remember: your worth isn't defined by your waistline, or a metric on anyone else's chart. After all, life's too short to be categorised by a nineteenth-century Belgian who never met you.

Sumo wrestlers

Bodies are like books: we should never judge them by their covers. Over the years, I've had the privilege (or burden) of examining and peering in to the abdomens of thousands of patients. I've seen people who would normally be considered overweight to have excellent blood markers for inflammation, lipids, blood glucose, cholesterol and extremely low levels of visceral fat internally. Conversely I could count a similar number of seemingly lean individuals with dangerously high levels of intra-abdominal fat and cholesterol levels, as well as other blood markers associated with poor metabolic health.

External appearances and 'vanity' metrics aren't everything. Sometimes, the answers lie beneath the superficial subcutaneous fat.

Take a sumo wrestler, for example. These larger-than-life gladiators might appear to be 'unhealthy', given the amount of food they consume and the degree of fat they carry. Granted, most people with obesity will store a higher amount of visceral fat deep in the body where it swaddles internal organs. Many sumo wrestlers, however, have far less visceral fat than a person of a similar size who doesn't throw opponents to the mat as a profession. In fact, they may even have lower levels of visceral fat than the average person too, despite their size. So what's the magic behind this?

CT scans have revealed that sumo wrestlers tend to carry subcutaneous fat. Typically, they also have normal blood lipid levels and unusually low cholesterol levels given their size and weight. Such biology-defying health is down to the fact that they are elite athletes. As studies have shown, exercise, particularly intense exercise, can prevent the accumulation and build-up of visceral fat. This is because exercise increases the production of the hormone adiponectin, which plays a crucial role in removing glucose and fat from the bloodstream, placing them in subcutaneous fat rather than visceral fat.

In a sumo stable (a *heya*), wrestlers train for several hours each day. One of their exercises, known as *butsukari-geiko*, involves hitting, pushing and shoving each other until the point of exhaustion. This is then followed by training matches and more group exercises. To fuel this intensity, and build size and strength, sumo wrestlers can consume upwards of 7,000 calories per day, but just like any elite-level athlete, once they retire, a sumo wrestler needs to reduce their calorie consumption in order to lower their risk of cardiovascular disease.

Weight loss weirdness

Body fat in women

Is it good for a woman to have a six-pack? The answer is nuanced and isn't served by a binary response. On average, women have a higher essential body fat percentage than men at 12 per cent versus around 3 per cent. This is biologically driven because body fat plays a key role in oestrogen production. Low oestrogen can negatively affect mood, sleep quality and bone density, and can disrupt menstruation and reproductive health.

Having a period is a metabolically demanding process. If your body is burning through energy to keep up with exercise or cope with stress, poor sleep and extreme dieting, it may need to conserve energy. One way to do this is to shut down ovulation and stop menstruation. Put in another way, the biological purpose of a menstrual cycle is to lay the groundwork for a potential pregnancy. If the body's fuel supply is low, the body interprets it as not a safe time to have a baby, so it will remove the need for menstruation.

For most women, striving for a body fat percentage low enough to reveal abs or a six-pack is not necessarily healthy. In fact, post-menopausal women who have a lowered oestrogen level would probably benefit from a higher body fat percentage to offset the rate of bone density loss and disruption to metabolic health. Ultimately, a six-pack isn't the true marker of health, either physically or mentally. It's also worth noting that fat distribution anatomically is also genetically driven so one person can have visible abs at a higher body fat than someone else.

DODGY DIETS

Let me begin by holding up my hands and levelling with you: there is no such thing as a miracle weight-loss programme beyond the combination of a balanced diet and a regular exercise programme. I am well aware that my voice is likely to be drowned out by the seductive claims made by the weight-loss industry, who profit from rendering fat as a social taboo. I just have to rely on the fact that I have science to back me up like some meat-head bouncer, and you're not going to be fooled, right?

What is the best diet?

You might find yourself drowning in the sea of bestselling nutrition and diet books, overwhelmed by the menagerie of weight-loss advice on social media or overburdened by the density of fat-shedding tips and tricks in magazines and newspapers. Despite this apparent wealth of information, no diet practitioners or self-styled weight-loss gurus can agree on the ultimate nutritional deliverance. Sometimes it's tempting to ignore the noise and just eat something that tastes damn good.

It's well established that improvements in the quality of our diet are associated with improvements in lifespan and healthspan as well as a decline in risk of many chronic diseases. Even so, there continues to be an argument as to what constitutes the best diet. The zealots promise the most with the least amount of evidence and often are polarising in their food choices and recommendations. To me, these people often represent potentially dangerous ideologies that can worsen people's relationship with food and even drive eating disorders.

I genuinely do not care which diet is best. I care about sustainability in a person's life. Even though I would include my life in this equation, I don't have a dog in this nutritional race. With no diet plan to shove down your throat, hopefully that means I can shine an unbiased, science-based take on the subject.

Saying that, I do have personal experience of the subject and have fallen prey to many a diet fad over the years, from low-carb to vegan to paleo and various others. Despite how prevalent these diets are on social media and in our culture, there remains a notable lack of long-term studies using rigorous methodology to back them up.

Where most diet zealots fail is the refusal to accept the energy-balance model, a fundamental law of thermodynamics that simply states that if you consume more energy in the form of calories than you burn, you will gain weight. As we will come to explore, there are some nuances that can be added to this equation, which can make the energy balance difficult due to various psychological, behavioural, societal, financial, physical, microbiome-related or disease-associated factors, but ultimately the equation remains true.

I'd argue that there is no one-size-fits-all 'best diet'. Instead, there are common denominators across eating patterns that are universally beneficial to your health. In very broad strokes, a diet that is high in fibre, high in minimally processed foods and predominantly plant-based, with a variety of food groups, appears to be associated with the best chance of disease prevention and good health.

Fads

Often a new diet craze gains prominence and then fizzles out just as quickly as it was introduced: raw food, detox, paleo – the list goes on. Ultimately, these quick fixes are ineffective because they prioritise short-term changes that fail to address long-term sustainable habits. The severe stringency and restriction of certain types of foods in these diets aren't sustainable and often come with the risk of nutritional deficiency and lack of any rigorous scientific evidence. Let's look at a few of the more popular diet fads.

Raw food diet

Raw food proponents claim that cooking destroys nutrients and vitamins in food. While cooking does degrade some nutrition, it also destroys any harmful micro-organisms in food so it is safer to eat and easier to digest, enabling our gut to absorb more of the nutrients.

Cooking doesn't just make food more palatable; it's nature's way of unlocking hidden treasures that your raw carrot sticks can only dream of. Through the alchemy of heat, cell walls break down, chemical bonds shift and previously inaccessible nutrients are unleashed, ready to be absorbed and put to good use by your body. Here are some prime examples of nutrients that cooking helps to unlock:

- **Lycopene (tomatoes):** Lycopene is a carotenoid pigment with potent antioxidant properties. Heating tomatoes significantly increases their lycopene content by breaking down cell walls, making this antioxidant more readily absorbed. So tomato sauces, roasted tomatoes, or even ketchup (yes, ketchup can be functional if not sugar-laden).

- **Beta-carotene (carrots, sweet potatoes, squash):** A precursor to vitamin A, beta-carotene is crucial for vision, immune function and skin health. Cooking carrots and other beta-carotene-rich foods enhances absorption by softening plant cell walls and dissolving it into fats when cooked with oils. Vitamin A deficiency can lead to night blindness and weakened immunity. Roast, steam, or sauté carrots and sweet potatoes in olive oil for maximum benefit.

- **Polyphenols (spinach, kale, broccoli):** Polyphenols are antioxidants that reduce inflammation and support heart health. Polyphenols are linked to reduced risk of chronic diseases like diabetes and cancer. Light steaming or sautéing greens often improves the release of polyphenols while retaining their nutrients.

The paleo diet

In 2012, Google Trends showed a sharp rise in searches for the 'paleo diet', which is often called the 'caveman diet'. This diet fad urged people to consume food as our ancestors did in the Palaeolithic era (which lasted from about 2.6 million years ago to 10,000 BC), claiming this was more aligned with our natural biology. This diet focuses on whole foods – fruits, vegetables, lean meat, nuts, eggs and seeds – which all sounds great. However, it omits whole grains and legumes, which are excellent sources of fibre and rich in essential nutrients and vitamins.

Strict adherence to diets like paleo – without a medical reason or allergy – can lead to nutritional deficiencies. And when you consider that ancient humans ate whatever was available, including on occasion other humans and other questionable items – the modern diet doesn't quite stack up to its name.

The keto diet and carbohydrates

Having tried many diets over the years, this one in particular not only made me miserable (even though I did lose weight, which was my goal), but also caused an extreme blockage of my internal plumbing.

The keto or ketogenic diet was originally developed as a way to help manage epilepsy in children. Over time it morphed into a belief system that designated carbohydrate-rich foods as inherently 'bad' and proposed a diet that recommended high healthy fat intake but very low carbohydrate consumption.

Most proponents of the keto diet have twisted the science to claim that the reason the diet improves metabolic health and causes weight loss is that a scarcity of carbs means less insulin secretion. Without insulin signalling to the body that it should focus on incoming glucose (from the carbs) it instead turns to fat stores.

Science, however, tells a different story. While keto can lead to initial weight loss, a significant portion of that is water loss not fat loss. In fact, low-carb diets are no more effective than high-carb diets for fat loss when calories are matched.

I can't completely malign the keto diet – for some people it certainly has its merits. As I experienced, it can be effective for short-term weight loss, largely because cutting out carbohydrates often means cutting out refined, heavily processed foods like white bread, sweets and crisps. These tend to be nutrient poor, hypercaloric and hyperpalatable, leading to a cycle of overeating and not feeling satisfied.

This Is Vital Information

Low-carb diets like keto can work in the short term but after about a year their effectiveness tends to match that of other diets. After just three months of minimising my carbohydrate intake, I saw decent shifts in my weight alongside severe constipation, but my gut and brain hungered for carbs daily and as I approached the eight to nine month mark, it became totally unsustainable.

Plant-based diets

If carbs truly were the enemy and a macronutrient that we should exclude from our diets, then vegetarians and vegans should be shaking in their hemp-laced boots. But they aren't.

Before continuing, I must make an admission that I am neither vegetarian nor vegan (however, I have tried both), and so when I offer a positive analysis of these diets, it is without bias or conflicts of interest – unless enjoying plant-based food qualifies as a conflict of interest, in which case I am biased as hell.

Large-scale epidemiological studies suggest that a high-carb diet of plant-based foods is associated with lower body weight, BMI and risk of chronic diseases. In fact, one large study of more than 800,000 individuals showed that vegetarianism and veganism led to a 15–21 per cent risk reduction in cardiovascular disease. Carbohydrates have an essential role in diets and many fibre-rich foods happen to be carb-rich, like legumes, and lentils in particular.

> *Note for vegans*
>
> If you follow a vegan diet without supplements, it is wise to be aware of your intake of key nutrients like vitamin B12 and iron, which are found in greater amounts in animal products. This is because iron found in plant food (non-heme iron) is less well absorbed than heme iron found in

meats (a rate of 1–10 per cent absorption of non-heme iron vs 20–40 per cent absorption for heme iron).

Dietary guidelines usually recommend that vegans aim for 1.8 times the recommended daily intake of iron for non-vegans. The good news, however, is that long-term vegans develop better absorption efficiency over time (up to 40 per cent improvement).

How to boost iron absorption naturally

- **Pair iron with vitamin C:** 75mg of vitamin C (about one orange) can significantly boost iron absorption
- **Time tea/coffee and any iron-rich meals:** Natural tannins found in your favourite hot beverage can reduce iron absorption, so leave a time gap between drinks and foods.

Here are some smart food pairings that will help with iron absorption:

- **Breakfast:** Oatmeal + strawberries (vitamin C) = absorption boost
- **Lunch:** Lentil soup + tomato (vitamin C) = absorption boost
- **Dinner:** Tofu stir fry + bell peppers (vitamin C) = absorption boost
- **Daily iron goal:** 1.8 x RDA (32mg women/ 14mg men).

Things I wish people knew about nutrition and diets

- **The best diet is a simple one you can stick to consistently.** As Michael Pollan said: 'Eat food. Not too much. Mostly plants.' Think less about restricting your diet, and more about what you can ADD to it and what you can GAIN. Your eating pattern should not follow a cookie-cutter recipe but rather be tailored to your lifestyle and your preferences.

This Is Vital Information

- **Unpopular opinion but nonetheless true; any diet can cause weight loss.** A sandwich-only diet, a McDonald's-only diet(!), a salmon-only diet. You get the point. This is true as long as there is some deficit created. In terms of weight loss, the actual diet itself makes little difference, but there are way more important health metrics beyond just weight in isolation.

- **Severe dietary restrictions are often the enemy of long-term goals.** Not only can they invoke nutrient deficiencies due to limited variety but they can promote disordered eating behaviours and affect your mood.

- **When you hear the word 'detox' when a diet is mentioned, run for the hills.** This is an important red flag to spot pseudoscientific terminology and the beginning of another fad.

- **Protein is key for muscle-buiding and maintenance, but you probably don't need as much as you think.** The minimum amount of protein to avoid ill-health should be 1g per kilogram of body weight per day. If you're over sixty-five or in peri/post-menopause, look at consuming 1.2g/kg/day; if you're pregnant or lactating 1.3g/kg/day appears to be a good target; if you're experiencing rapid weight loss aim for 1.4g/kg/day; if you're experiencing rapid weight loss and you're increasing activity aim for 1.6g/kg/day. A basic formula to follow goes something like this: your weight (kg) x g/kg/day = target (g). It's also worth noting that protein needs to rise with activity, so from low activity to moderate, high, strength training or for athletes, it can increase from 1, 1.2, 1.4, 1.6 to 2g/kg/day respectively. While you might hear some complexities touted about having a certain amount of protein per meal, the vagaries matter not. What's more important is your total protein load across a twenty-four-hour period. And yes, all plants contain all twenty amino acids, including the nine essential ones, so eating a variety of plant-based foods ensures you get them all.

- **Gluten isn't bad for you *unless* you have coeliac disease or non-coeliac gluten sensitivity or a gluten allergy.** If you don't fall into any of these brackets and you've found anecdotally that avoiding gluten makes you feel better or minimises any negative symptoms, by all means give it a miss, but there is no objective evidence suggesting a gluten-free diet for the average person is better than a gluten-inclusive diet. In fact, there is some data suggesting it could have adverse health outcomes such as nutrient deficiency due to a decreased consumption of whole grains, which are generally associated with positive health effects. Moreover, gluten-free foods are way more expensive, so the biggest effect will be on your bank balance.

- **Diets don't have to be complex.** There are some basics worth adhering to no matter what dietary religion you happen to be following:

    a) Overconsumption of most things will follow the rule of diminishing returns to a point where it becomes negative. Same goes with calories. Calorie restriction has anti-inflammatory potential.

    b) Food diversity in type, variety and colour is almost always beneficial. There is some merit to the phrase 'Taste the rainbow' (even though the original Starburst advert may not be the ideal food to analogise this). Different colours = different types of plant chemicals (phytonutrients, flavonoids and antioxidants), which are all anti-inflammatory in nature.

    c) Everyone knows less fried food = better health, and minimising your saturated fat is advisable. Having said this, having some fried chicken or French fries once in a while (not every day, mind) isn't going to be the death of you.

This Is Vital Information

CELLULITE: THE DIMPLED LEGACY OF ANATOMY, CAPITALISM AND CULTURAL NEUROSES

If you've ever caught sight of the dimples on your thighs, you might've wondered when your legs started impersonating a golf ball. Rest assured, you're not alone, and it's not a defect. It's cellulite, the unwitting star of one of history's longest-running scams. How did a benign, completely normal anatomical variation become the scourge of Instagram filters and the foundation of a multibillion-dollar industry?

The word 'cellulite' first slinked on to the scene in 1873 in a French medical dictionary. Back then, it was a benign term to describe fat deposits beneath the skin – just biology doing its thing.

For decades it stayed in obscurity, lurking quietly in dermatological texts. Then came the twentieth century, and with it, the beauty industry's knack for inventing problems to sell solutions. In the 1960s, European beauty salons began using the term 'cellulite' in marketing materials, reframing it not as a natural occurrence but as a cosmetic flaw, a scourge that women should battle with the ferocity of a medieval knight slaying a dragon. By the time *Vogue* introduced cellulite to American readers in the 1970s, it had morphed from medical jargon to a full-blown crisis.

In anatomical terms, cellulite is subcutaneous fat pressing against the connective tissue beneath the skin, creating a dimpled, uneven surface. It's not a disease. It's not a toxin build-up. It's just fat interacting with fibrous septae, which are connective tissue bands that tether the skin to underlying structures.

Women's skin has a vertical arrangement of connective tissue, which makes it easier for fat to push through and create dimples. Men's connective tissue forms a criss-cross pattern, offering a sturdier 'net' that keeps fat in check.

Women naturally store more fat in areas like the thighs and buttocks due to hormonal influences, particularly oestrogen, making it more likely that they will have cellulite. In fact, 80–90 per cent of women have cellulite. It's so common it might as well be a secondary sex characteristic. Fluctuations in oestrogen can weaken connective tissue and exacerbate cellulite's appearance. Men don't escape entirely, but their cellulite prevalence is far lower.

By the mid-twentieth century, cellulite had become a sociocultural villain, fed by shifting beauty ideals, patriarchy and new fashions such as miniskirts and sheer tights, which put skin on display.

The end result was the birth of the anti-cellulite industry, which now rakes in billions annually. Creams, massages, lasers, and even DIY treatments like coffee scrubs have flooded the market, each promising to 'banish' cellulite. P.S., they don't.

Most cellulite treatments are glorified snake oil, supported by marketing hyperbole rather than science. Anti-cellulite creams? These usually contain caffeine or retinol, which may temporarily tighten the skin by dehydrating it. But does this fix cellulite? No. It's like putting concealer on a cracked wall and ignoring the structural issue.

What about massages and lymphatic drainage? These techniques claim to reduce cellulite by improving circulation. While they might temporarily reduce puffiness, they don't alter the underlying fat or connective tissue.

OK, but surely lasers and radiofrequency treatments work? High-tech devices promise to break down fat and tighten skin. Some show mild, temporary improvements, but the results rarely justify the cost.

If you're determined to tackle cellulite, here are some suggestions more grounded in reality:

- **Strength training:** Building muscle can improve skin tone and reduce the appearance of dimples by creating a firmer layer beneath the skin
- **Healthy lifestyle:** A balanced diet and regular exercise won't erase cellulite but can reduce fat stores, making it less noticeable

- **Laser-assisted procedures:** Medical treatments can improve cellulite by cutting the fibrous bands causing dimples. These kind of work, but they're expensive and not permanent.

But the most effective 'cure' for cellulite is acceptance. It's not a defect. It's part of being human, just like stretch marks, freckles, and that inexplicable urge to Google symptoms at midnight.

I BLAME SOCIETY

'You're fat because you're lazy.' So goes the argument for a surprising number of people who cannot fathom the complexity of what causes obesity. Obesity is usually defined as an excessive build-up of adipocytes or fat (defined as a BMI over thirty – but you know my reservations about BMI.

Obesity goes beyond willpower and 'eating too much'. There are numerous nuances that can influence someone's risk of obesity, including genetic factors such as a mutation in the FTO gene (meaning an abnormal increase in ghrelin levels). Environmental factors like the availability of food or even psychological factors such as childhood trauma can also predispose someone to disordered eating habits and binge eating.

One of the most important steps in changing the health of people across the globe is the food environment and food policy, and this requires change from on high.

Even in hospital settings, which are seen as beacons of improving health and cures, we are let down by food choices made available to us. A typical meal found in a hospital canteen consists of indeterminate slop layered with oil, or else a deep-fried piece of meat with overcooked chips; all available for a price far cheaper than the more nutritious options (if you're lucky enough to have them).

Even with an understanding of the nuances of obesity, we are shackled by the choices available to us. Governments and food manufacturers need to address the root problem and make healthy, nutrient-dense food cheaper and more accessible and more equitable rather than shifting blame and responsibility to the end consumer alone.

For all our moralising about personal responsibility when it comes to obesity, we're still missing the obvious. The problem isn't just individuals; it's the system – the insidious labyrinth of cheap junk food, predatory marketing, and a public health infrastructure that treats healthy eating as a luxury reserved for the Gwyneth Paltrows of this world.

If obesity were a chess game, we've been yelling at the pawns while letting the kings (governments) and queens (food corporations) run rampant. And we're losing the game.

Blaming individuals is easy. It's tidy. It makes for great soundbites like: 'Calories in, calories out!' or 'Just eat less and move more!' Never mind that these phrases have about as much practical use as yelling: 'Just swim!' to someone drowning in a riptide.

The choices we make are shaped by the choices we're given. If you're trying to buy nutrient-dense food but live in a food desert where the nearest broccoli is two bus rides away while a family-sized bag of crisps costs less than a single apple, what do you think is going to happen?

What if, instead of shaming people for choosing unhealthy options, we made healthy options the default? Governments and policymakers have a unique ability to shape the environment we live in, nudging the population towards better health outcomes without wagging a single accusatory finger. This is no pipe dream; such public health measures have worked in the past.

The UK soft drinks industry levy (aka the sugar tax), introduced in 2018, is a shining example of how policy can work. It slapped a tax on sugary drinks, incentivising manufacturers to reformulate their products with less sugar. By 2020, the sugar content in soft drinks had fallen by 35 per cent, cutting overall sugar consumption by hundreds of millions of kilograms annually. The £300 million-plus raised annually has been used to fund health initiatives, including school sports programmes.

Remember trans fats? The artery-clogging imposters that turned margarine and fried foods into little time bombs for your heart? In 2003, Denmark became the first country to ban trans fats outright. The results were staggering. Denmark saw a significant drop in cardiovascular mortality rates, proving that taking harmful substances off the shelves works better than asking people to read microscopic nutrition labels. Other countries followed suit, and in 2018, the World Health Organization (WHO) called for a worldwide ban on industrially produced trans fats.

Countries like Finland have shown that subsidising healthy foods can work wonders. By reducing the price of fruits and vegetables, Finland managed to increase their consumption and improve overall dietary quality, proving that accessibility is key.

The solutions seem obvious, so it is staggering that every government hasn't jumped on board. The food industry spends billions convincing policymakers that it's not junk food making people unhealthy, it's people making 'bad choices', despite having spent decades engineering products to be addictive enough to make heroin seem simply 'more-ish'.

If governments truly want to tackle obesity, here would be my suggested playbook:

- **Make healthy food affordable and accessible:** Subsidise fresh produce. Build supermarkets in food deserts. Make healthy eating less of a privilege and more of a right

- **Tax the bad stuff:** Sugar taxes, junk food levies and stricter advertising restrictions aren't just punitive. They work. And if companies complain, just remind them they're still turning a profit

- **Provide information:** Nutrition labels are nice, but they need to be clear, concise and backed by campaigns that actually resonate (nobody reads the fine print when they're hungry)

- **Regulate the industry:** Cap portion sizes, reduce salt and sugar content, and ban marketing to kids. If Denmark can do it, so can everyone else.

Obesity isn't just a personal issue, it's a collective one. In the end, food is more than fuel; it's culture, comfort and connection. Policies that make healthy eating easier don't just improve waistlines, they enrich lives. And that, surely, is worth a little corporate whining. Because if we can't fix a system that prioritises profits over people, maybe we deserve to be stuck with kale smoothies and sugar-free misery. Or we can dream a little bigger, aim a little higher, and remind the world that health isn't just an individual goal – it's a shared responsibility.

This Is Vital Information

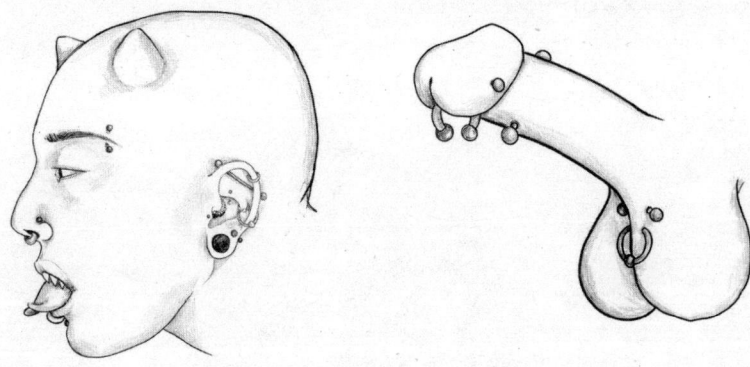

The modified human

Chapter 7

BODY MOD MAYHEM

I'VE SPENT MANY YEARS DOCUMENTING the family histories of thousands of patients. Each time, my aim is to decipher whether someone is at risk of a certain type of disease or condition, or to uncover clues that could lead to a diagnosis. In the same way, I've always been fascinated by my own family history and what it might reveal about me.

I'm not alone in this curiosity – you only need to look at the exponential growth of ancestry websites and DNA tests that can unlock your archaeological footprint from the comfort of your own home. For many cultures, however, their family histories are not transcribed on paper, but rather displayed on their skin or bodies.

Since the dawn of time, humans have used their bodies as a canvas for art, identity and self-expression. To fulfil this desire, they might get a tattoo, pierce holes in their bodies, or undergo surgery in a bid to enhance or alter their appearance. Body modification – by which we mean the deliberate altering of the body, usually for non-medical reasons – can also encompass more invasive practices: foot binding, lip plates and subdermal implants. These modifications push the boundaries of human creativity and are limited only by human imagination, and the body's capacity for pain.

This Is Vital Information

OTZI THE ICEMAN

In 1991, two German hikers ascending the Alps close to the Italian–Austrian border happened upon a frozen corpse in the ice. But this was no ordinary body. It was that of Otzi the Iceman, the nickname for a person who had died almost 5,300 years ago.

Further analysis of the frozen mummy revealed that he had dozens of tattoo-like marks all over his body – possibly the earliest evidence we have of tattooing. Many of these tattoos centred around his ankles, knees and spine, areas which, as X-rays revealed, showed signs of arthritis. The tattoos, which coincided with the acupuncture points for pain, may have been used to relieve pain in some way.

The word tattoo is believed to stem from the Tahitian 'tatau', which means to mark or strike the skin. It refers to the traditional Polynesian method of marking ink into the skin using a tool made of animal bone or sticks. Natural substances like burned ash or fungi were then placed into the wound, which would heal and form a permanent tattoo. When European explorers came face to face with these inked warriors and Polynesian tribes, the word and the act of tattooing caught on and eventually spread around the globe.

This is a world far removed from your local tattoo parlour, where artists use rotary needle guns that oscillate rapidly over the skin and penetrate to a depth of a mere 1mm to deliver pigments.

The end result is somewhat similar in a biological sense. Any pigment that finds its way into the inner sanctums of the body – in this case, the dermis (or middle layer of skin) – is treated as a foreign body, which needs to be contained. The macrophage cells of your immune system gather round the microscopic pigment particles, which are too big to be engulfed, unlike bacterial or viral units. Instead, they are surrounded and encapsulated by the ever-watchful macrophages and become fixed in the connective tissue of the dermis.

Body mod mayhem

Alongside icemen, tattoos have made regular appearances throughout history – just about every human culture around the world has been partial to inking. The ancient Greeks used tattoos as a form of espionage and communication, while the Romans employed them as a tool of control and punishment, branding slaves and criminals with permanent ink. A similar practice existed in early Japan, where criminals received a line tattooed on their forehead for each offence – one line for the first crime, two for the second, etc. – an early version of three strikes and you're out. Tattoos haven't been used only for punitive purposes. They have been used in ceremonies, to commemorate loved ones, mark status, or rites of passage, or to symbolise affiliation with a group or family.

In some parts of the world, tattoos have carried a social stigma. In the eighteenth and nineteenth centuries, tattoos in the Western world were associated with sailors, criminals and other outsiders, a perception that persisted well into the twentieth century, when they became linked to gang culture and biker communities.

The taboo surrounding tattooing is a little ironic considering the words 'tattoo' and 'taboo' not only sound similar but are derived from Polynesian languages (taboo from 'tapu', referring to something that is prohibited or sacred in Tongan and Māori).

These days the coolest celebrities sport body art and they've moved from a subcultural practice to a mainstream trend and a normalised form of self-expression. And yet, while tattoos have had quite the journey and they've certainly become more acceptable, there are still some quarters of society that look down on them. It seems they'll never be free from taboo.

The surgeon with ink

I worked with a surgeon a few years ago who was heavily inked up. When wearing his scrub top you could see his story written on his skin; the intricate pigmented whorls decorated his arms all the way to his wrists, with unique patterns poking out from the V-neck of his scrub to the throat.

This Is Vital Information

The tattoos were intimidating yet beautiful. One weekday morning, we were both in adjacent clinic rooms seeing patients. A nurse hurriedly entered my room and whispered to me, almost as if ashamed: 'The next patient doesn't want to see the other doctor. Could you see her, please?'

Slightly confused, I agreed, even if just to reduce my colleague's workload. I enquired as to why she didn't want to see him. The patient replied: 'He's obviously not very professional – doctors shouldn't have tattoos!'

That particular patient clearly felt she couldn't trust my colleague, preferring her doctors to have more of a conservative look, one that spoke of years of serious study, not of headlining Glastonbury.

My first tattoo

Of course, these days surgeons are not just sporting tattoos but using them in various forms of surgery. Several years ago, my boss and I were scheduled to perform a number of breast cancer operations. The list included a mastectomy for cancer (removing the entire breast), a wide local excision for cancer (removing a lump of cancerous breast tissue) . . . and nipple tattoos.

I asked my boss if there was a mistake on the list.

'No. You're going to do your first tattoo today,' he said. 'I'll show you!'

The patient in need of nipple tattoos had undergone a mastectomy several months earlier, which meant her nipples and areolas had departed too. In such cases, some people opt for nipple reconstruction, and these can offer good cosmetic outcomes. Reconstructed nipples, however, rarely look like the originals, typically lack sensation and often lose their shape and vertical projection, flattening over time.

As a result, this patient had chosen to go for 3D tattooed nipples. So, guided by my boss and summoning up the embers of creative and artistic flair deep within me, I set upon the task. Using a tattoo pen and a palette of inks to create highlights and shadowing, I managed – if I say so myself – to create amazingly realistic nipples, which appeared to have the illusion of depth. In the end, this was probably one of my proudest moments in surgery because it was so far removed from what I usually do, and potentially brought something positive to a patient who had been through such a difficult time.

Tattoo removal

Tattoos and regret are long-lost friends. If you choose to get a tattoo, you may love it for ever or come to regret permanently inking yourself with the name of a former flame, that leaping tiger that now looks a little more stretched, or a sobering reminder of a drunken night out. Whatever the reason, once you decide a tattoo must go, the most common and effective method is by laser removal.

You might think a laser simply zaps the tattoo and it disappears but, in fact, the process is a little more complicated . . .

When you are first marked with ink, the tattoo needle pushes a big chunk of ink into the dermis layer of the skin, where your immune cells lurk. Your white blood cells (specifically macrophages) view the ink particles as foreign bodies and the greedy b******s try to gobble them up in one go (picture a mouse trying to take a bite out of an elephant).

The white blood cells have some degree of success, which explains why tattoos fade slightly over time but what really helps is a laser using pulses of concentrated light to shatter the ink pigments into smaller, 'bite size' pieces. The hungry white cells then gradually flush them out through the lymphatic system.

Eventually, the majority of these ink particles are removed via defecation, urination and sweat. Yes, that's right, you poop out your tattoo. However, I will caveat this by saying that the tattoo ink will not be visible in your excrement so please do not go looking for it.

Pierce of mind

Growing up in the 1990s and early 2000s, my parents never had to worry that teenage angst would drive me to get a piercing.

Given the increasing influence of piercings in pop culture – Britney Spears, Limp Bizkit, Christina Aguilera, and even the nipple piercing seen in Janet Jackson's 'nip-slip' during the Super Bowl half-time show in 2004 – I was probably something of an anomaly. I was just never aesthetically attracted to piercings, nor did I ever want to have another one.

Yes, I said 'another one' because I already had my ears pierced.

When I was a newborn, as is popular in Indian culture, I had my ears pierced as part of a practice known in Sanskrit as Karna Vedha, a tradition that has deep cultural and religious roots. In Hinduism, ear piercing is considered one of the sixteen samskaras, sacred rites of passage that mark important stages in a person's life. The Karna Vedha is believed to help purify the body and mind and prepare the child for a prosperous, virtuous life, while also providing protection from evil spirits and negative energies. I had my ears pierced in a temple in India (under sterile conditions, I assume) and was adorned with earrings until I was around three years old.

I no longer wear an earring (I haven't since I was two years old) and over the years my body has filled in the holes, but I can still feel the tiny hollows where the piercings once were. I don't plan to re-pierce them or continue the tradition with my future children . . . unless, of course, they grow up and want to punch holes in their own bodies.

Piercings are by no means a modern invention. They have a strong cultural and spiritual history spanning thousands of years and across many cultures.

Our friend Otzi the Iceman had pierced ears and the Ancient Egyptians, Greeks and Romans all practised ear piercing often as a sign of rank or wealth. In Indian culture, nose piercing signifies marital status and in tribal cultures of the Americas, Africa and Oceania, lip and tongue piercing has been practised for various aesthetic, social and spiritual purposes. Genital pierces have been used to enhance sexual pleasure or as a rite of passage, and were utilised in Ancient Rome to prevent slaves from procreating.

Despite their ubiquity today, piercings still raise eyebrows, especially when they venture beyond the ears. A tasteful stud on the lobe? Classy. But show up with a septum ring or a bar through your eyebrow, and suddenly Aunt Mildred can't stop clutching her pearls.

Humans are hardwired to be wary of anything that deviates from the norm. Especially if that deviation involves sharp objects with seemingly sexual undertones (I'm looking at you, nipple and genital piercings). And anything remotely connected to sex has been taboo since, well, for ever.

The Prince Albert

On the topic of genital piercings, I'd be remiss if I didn't bring up the Prince Albert – a piercing that's as infamous as it is misunderstood. For the uninitiated, this is a male genital piercing that involves inserting jewellery through the underside of the penis and out through the opening of the urethra. Legend (almost certainly apocryphal) has it that the piercing was named after Queen Victoria's husband, Prince Albert, who allegedly used it to fasten his genitals to his trousers.

Why do men get a Prince Albert? Reasons range from aesthetic appeal to enhanced pleasure for both the wearer and their partner.

Healing takes six to eight weeks, during which you'll become intimately familiar with the phrase 'gentle handling'. Obviously, such a delicate piercing isn't without risks, including urinary tract infections (because you're putting a foreign object through your urethra), scarring or complications if not done properly.

The process of piercing

All piercings, wherever they are on the body, are a type of medical procedure because they involve creating a wound, which must heal and needs aftercare.

This Is Vital Information

After any wound, healing begins with the inflammatory stage, during which the area may feel tender and appear raw as the immune system gathers the cavalry to rush to the site of exposure.

Next comes the proliferative or growth phase. The supply chains of the body begin to take shape as cells and proteins are manufactured to heal the puncture site and the skin edges pucker or contract eventually, forming a more controlled open wound known as a fistula. This stage can last weeks if not months.

Finally, during the remodelling or maturation stage, the wound strengthens and stabilises. During the healing process it is perfectly normal to see discharge, which is often sebum, an oily substance produced by the sebaceous glands to keep the area moisturised.

When piercings go wrong

For all their beauty and cultural significance, piercings come with risks. Your body isn't always thrilled about being punctured, and when things go wrong, it's less 'self-expression' and more 'biohazard'.

Rejection occurs when the body decides your piercing is an intruder and tries to push it out like a bad Tinder match. Signs include the jewellery moving closer to the surface of the skin, redness, swelling and tenderness (beyond the normal healing period) and the area looking like it's dressed up for a medical drama.

If you notice any of this then remove any jewellery and avoid reinserting it until the area is fully healed. Your body isn't a pin-cushion and if the rejection persists, consult a healthcare provider.

Improper aftercare or unsterilised equipment can also lead to infections. You may notice persistent pain, redness or warmth around the site, discharge (especially if it's yellow or green), and fever or chills (a rare but serious sign the infection is spreading).

In such instances, clean the piercing with saline solution – not vodka,

Body mod mayhem

no matter what TikTok says — and avoid touching it with dirty hands. If symptoms worsen you should seek medical attention as antibiotics may be needed.

> To avoid problems with piercings, my advice is to:
>
> - **Opt for high-quality jewellery.** It could be made of surgical steel, titanium or gold, and if a reaction occurs, switch to hypoallergenic materials immediately. Many cheaper metals contain nickel, which is notorious for causing allergic reactions. Symptoms include itching, redness and an angry rash that makes you question your life choices.
>
> - **Choose a reputable piercer.** Go to someone who uses sterile equipment, wears gloves and ideally doesn't moonlight as a pirate. Make sure you stick to the aftercare instructions and avoid swimming during healing: chlorine and bacteria are not your friends. Just be patient. Healing takes time and rushing it is a surefire way to end up with regrets (and scars).

At their core, piercings are about identity. They're a way of claiming your body as your own in a world that's constantly trying to dictate what it should look like. Whether it's a discreet stud or a constellation of metalwork, piercings can be a subtle act of rebellion.

But they're also a reminder of our fragility. Skin breaks. Bodies reject. Healing takes time. And sometimes, the things we do to express ourselves come with complications. So, if your body rebels against your piercing, don't sweat it. Take it out, clean it up, and remember: your worth isn't measured by the holes you keep but by the confidence you wear, whether or not there's a Prince Albert involved.

SCARIFICATION

Scars can mean all manner of things. For many, they are a permanent reminder that we are all clumsy dumbasses. Others purposely harm themselves as a means of expressing or numbing difficult feelings, a mental health issue that can be treated. Then there are those who deliberately create scars on the skin for aesthetic, spiritual or personal reasons. This is scarification, which involves cutting, etching or branding the skin in specific patterns or shapes, practised in various cultures around the world as well as in modern society as an alternative to tattoos or as a form of self-expression.

In Papua New Guinea's East Sepik region, scarification remains a rite of passage for young boys becoming men. The riverside 'spirit houses', or Haus Tambaran, foster a local belief system that deifies animals like the crocodile. To imbue bestial power, the young boys and men of the East Sepik have their bodies cut by razor blades and sharpened bamboo to leave raised scars that resemble crocodile teeth and skin. In Ethiopia's Karo tribe, marks on the men's chests can signify they have killed a dangerous animal or enemy, whereas raised scars on girls may indicate they have gone through puberty or are ready for marriage.

Scars in all their forms, through ritual scarification, surgery or as a result of injury, tell the world of your past. An archive written on your skin. So how exactly are they formed?

Imagine that while turning a page of this book, you give yourself the most agonising of minor injuries: a paper cut. A trickle of blood oozes from the fine incision. What happens next is a meticulously choreographed process of healing and self-preservation. First, the bleeding is arrested during a process called haemostasis (from the Greek word 'haem' – blood – and 'stasis' – stop).

The cut blood vessels then immediately go into a brief spasm, narrowing to further stem the bleeding. Shortly after, the cavalry arrives in the form of platelets. These microscopic disc-like cells coalesce and stick to the damaged inner lining of the blood vessels, where they release a heady cocktail of immune molecules that trigger clotting. More platelets add to the expanding lump, plugging the wound and eventually forming a scab. It's a finely tuned symphony of healing that happens within the space of a few minutes.

Over the years I've seen thousands of scars, from tiny, almost unnoticeable marks on groin creases or forearms, to huge vertical scars splitting the mid-section of patients like a briefcase zipper signifying some major emergency abdominal operation. I've also seen the 'Mercedes-Benz' scar of patients who've had liver surgery, so called because it resembles the three-pointed star logo of a Mercedes car.

I've created scars, removed them, sliced through old ones and even done my best to avoid them, but the nature of my profession and the biological inevitability of wound-healing means that often a permanent mark on the skin is a done deal.

I've also collected a few scars of my own over the years, from foolish childhood adventures gone wrong (that's a book of its own) to accidents in everyday life, and although our scars are a manifestation of memories, regrets, choices and life experiences, we often try to hide or conceal them like a horrible secret.

Earlier in my career I saw a woman in her forties with a hernia poking through a C-section scar that needed fixing. I vividly remember her asking if I could also fix her C-section scar at the same time to make it 'go away' and 'more presentable'.

Of course, I understand that living with a scar can be difficult, yet some scars, although forged in pain, are a consequence of something astounding and in the case of a C-section scar the postscript of a new life.

With this in mind, there are some scientifically proven ways to 'improve' the appearance of any surgical wounds or scars you might have, both in the early and late stages.

This Is Vital Information

- **Moisturiser:** This encourages skin hydration, leading to a better wound in the early stages of scar formation, supporting tissue generation and cell migration. The more hydrated the skin is, the more 'plastic' or flexible it is, which can reduce the chances of a raised (hypertrophic) scar. Use a fragrance-free moisturiser.

- **Silicone gel:** This creates a thin protective layer over a wound, preventing water loss and redness, flattening and softening the scar tissue over time.

- **Sunscreen:** A dermatologist's best friend is surprisingly good for scars. During the wound-healing stage, the skin will be thinner and UV rays can also cause hyperpigmentation and worsen the appearance of scars by triggering melanin production in this healing tissue.

- **Massage:** This can improve blood flow, help to soften scar tissue and improve its overall appearance by regulating collagen deposition (too much of which can lead to raised scars). Gently massage the scar for ten minutes twice daily (but only once the wound has fully healed).

- **Retinoids:** This one needs to be directed by your doctor, but we know that retinoids help to increase the turnover of skin cells and promote collagen production. This can make scars smoother and prevent abnormal collagen accumulation.

- **Laser therapy:** Again, this should be overseen by a dermatologist but laser therapy can break down scar tissue and target the deeper layers of skin and help to improve both scar colour and texture.

- **Steroids:** No, not the body-building type, but corticosteroids can help to reduce inflammation and excess collagen accumulation and are especially effective for hypertrophic (enlarged) or keloid (a type of raised) scars.

- **Don't use bleach!** I really shouldn't have to say this, but don't use bleach to clean wounds. This is extremely caustic to wounds and can slow the healing process, resulting in a poor wound appearance.

- **Diet:** During wound healing there are certain components that are key for tissue regeneration, including sufficient protein intake for new cell production as well as nutrients like vitamins C and E, and zinc, which are all crucial for collagen synthesis.

PIMP MY RIDE

These days, self-expression has evolved into something far greater and expansive than our ancestors could ever have imagined. I'm not talking about piercing or scarring other parts of the body, but rather the new world of body modification.

Body modifications include not just tattoos and ear piercings but also more invasive procedures like tongue splitting, elf ears (sculpting the ear into a pointy shape), subdermal implants (inserting objects under the skin), removing parts of the body, injecting ink into the whites of the eyes, and removing or filing teeth, to name but a few.

These more esoteric procedures create an aesthetic that is well beyond the boundaries of 'normal' social constructs. The reasons why someone might decide to get their eyeballs tattooed or get a horn implant on their head are varied. They want to do more than stand out; they want to create a unique identity, use their body as a canvas for expression, or rebel against societal norms. Or in some rare cases could they be a sign of mental health issues?

Perhaps, in a way, body modifications help to bridge the gap between reality and fantasy. While I truly believe in self-expression and subscribe to the belief that everyone should do what they like to their own body – get a boob job if you must and pierce your nipples if that makes you happy. But I must also put my doctor's hat on and query whether people who undergo more extreme modifications are given appropriate counselling about the risks, side effects or the irreversibility of some of these procedures and the impact they may have on body function. Are the surgeons and artists who offer these 'out there' procedures looking after the best interests of their patients or their own bank balances?

Anyone practising body modifications should outline to prospective patients the psychological and physical consequences of certain procedures, whether it's subdermal implants or removing a rib – and it's also the duty of the practitioner to assess the pre-surgical well-being of the patient.

The ethics of amputations

In my early years as a surgical trainee, I was assisting a vascular surgeon in an emergency amputation. The patient had a case of necrotising fasciitis (aka flesh-eating disease) and the infection was rapidly spreading up his leg.

The patient was a smoker and a diabetic. He had had a small ulcer on his toe that became infected (which is common in diabetics due to their higher risk of infection). On arriving in A&E, he was almost unconscious with a barely palpable pulse. He also possessed a blackened, flaky, pus-ridden leg that resembled a piece of rotting wood.

The patient required an emergency below-knee amputation to limit the spread of infection. Over the next few days, as the infection returned like a weed that had survived pruning, he would return to theatre so we could continue chipping away at further bits of dead tissue that appeared at the base of the previous amputations.

The above patient didn't ask for this procedure but, as bizarre as it sounds, there are people who voluntarily request the removal of a normally functioning body part, forcing disability upon themselves.

Body integrity identity disorder

In 1875, French surgeon Jean-Joseph Sue found himself dealing with an English patient who had fallen in love with a one-legged woman. In order to win over his *amour* he wanted to amputate his own (perfectly good) leg.

So frenzied was his love that he held Dr Sue at gunpoint and demanded that his leg be removed. Sue, feeling he had no choice, agreed to the surgery. This was the first documented and subsequently published entry of body integrity identity disorder (BIID).

Thankfully, BIID is incredibly rare. It makes sufferers feel like a limb or part of their body doesn't belong to them and they develop a strong desire to amputate or disable the seemingly alien entity. BIID can also extend to senses, causing a thirty-year-old woman who reportedly believed she was meant to have been born blind to ask a psychologist to pour drain cleaner into her eyes to remove her sight.

It wasn't until the 1990s that researchers began to gain a better understanding of BIID. Research from that time suggested that it was associated with an abnormality in the right parietal lobe of the brain, which plays an important role in spatial awareness and a person's 'sense of self'.

Researchers found that those with BIID often show a reduction in the thickness of the right parietal lobe, which may cause feelings of disconnectedness to a body part so it no longer feels like it belongs to them.

Disturbingly, many BIID sufferers report feeling relief or a sense of completeness with their new disabilities. This behaviour might appear shocking to a casual observer but parallels have been drawn between BIID and body dysmorphic disorder (BDD) since both groups of patients have obsessions with parts of their bodies.

BDD is a mental health condition where individuals become excessively preoccupied with perceived flaws in their appearance, even if these flaws seem minor or non-existent to others. These concerns can lead to significant distress and impact greatly on daily life. Common symptoms include constant checking or avoiding mirrors, excessive grooming, seeking cosmetic procedures or avoidance of social situations due to anxiety over appearance.

While BDD involves distorted perceptions of one's physical appearance, BIID is feeling that a particular part of the body doesn't belong or is incongruous with one's self-image, despite it being physically healthy and functional. Both conditions can cause profound emotional distress but stem from different root causes and affect the body–mind connection in distinct ways. Crucially, someone with BDD feels as if a body part is flawed and requires improvement; for example, by seeking a 'nose job' for cosmetic purposes, rather than seeking to be liberated from the nose altogether, like those in Camp BIID.

Treating patients with BIID is extremely challenging and further complicated by the fact that psychotherapy is rarely successful. Most doctors have deep-seated moral and ethical qualms about removing healthy limbs from patients who want to become disabled. This is a perfect storm of bodily autonomy versus ethics, and the solution is far from straightforward.

This ethical dilemma came into sharp focus in January 2000 when it was widely reported in the media that Robert Smith, a surgeon working at the Falkirk and District Royal Infirmary in Scotland, had amputated the healthy legs of two patients at their request. The surgeon was criticised by the NHS trust that ran the hospital, which described these amputations as 'inappropriate'. Since 2000 no hospital in the UK has performed these voluntary amputations. The case underscored just how contentious and unresolved the issue remains – medically, morally and legally.

Can body modifications be good?

Body modification in all its forms is often seen primarily as a form of self-expression but it also serves an important and often overlooked role in the medical realm.

Medical body modifications are the unsung heroes of human ingenuity. They're where medicine meets engineering, with a splash of 'What if we added Bluetooth?' Today's innovations include bionic limbs that can be controlled by brain signals, allowing amputees to regain mobility and even a sense of touch.

Body mod mayhem

Prosthetics aren't just practical any more – they're works of art. From glow-in-the-dark arms to custom designs, they allow wearers to reclaim their identity while flipping the middle finger to stigma (literally, if the bionics are advanced enough).

Beyond limbs, devices like cochlear implants can help restore senses. These marvels of science restore hearing to those with profound hearing loss by bypassing damaged parts of the ear and directly stimulating the auditory nerve. Cochlear implants raise fascinating debates about identity. Some in the deaf community view them as eroding deaf culture, while others see them as tools of empowerment. Either way, they're proof that body modification can profoundly reshape our connection to the world.

From pacemakers to insulin pumps, implants save lives and improve quality of life. Imagine trying to convince someone in the 1800s that your heart beats thanks to a tiny machine. Witchcraft? Nope, just science.

Experimental devices like neural implants are already in development, promising everything from pain management to enhanced memory. We're edging closer to becoming actual cyborgs, which is both exhilarating and terrifying.

The blurred line between 'restoration' and 'enhancement' raises questions. If you're improving function *and* form, who's to say it's purely medical or purely aesthetic? (P.S., it's usually both.)

Of course, body modification, even for medical purposes, isn't without its risks. Your body is a notoriously finicky house guest: it doesn't always take kindly to foreign objects, no matter how high-tech they are. The risk of complications always remains – your body might reject implants, which can lead to inflammation, infection and the heartbreaking need to start over.

Medical or not, any time you introduce something foreign to the body, bacteria might get in on the act too. The solution? Meticulous hygiene and regular check-ups.

This Is Vital Information

Modern devices like pacemakers or insulin pumps rely on software, and, well, software can glitch. Imagine having to reboot your pancreas like it's a Windows 98 desktop.

If you're considering body modification for medical reasons, here's what to keep in mind:

- **Choose a trusted provider:** Whether it's a cochlear implant or a prosthetic limb, work with professionals who know their stuff. This is not the time to recoup a voucher for 50 per cent off from a backstreet surgeon.

- **Understand the risks:** Ask about rejection rates, infection risks and long-term maintenance. Pro tip: 'Will this beep at airport security?' is a valid question.

- **Keep it clean:** Whether it's a surgical implant or a dermal anchor (a metal base inserted just below the skin usually for body jewellery), hygiene is your best friend. If something looks or feels off, don't wait – call a doctor.

- **Think long-term:** Medical modifications are rarely 'set it and forget it'. Stay up-to-date on maintenance, replacements or software upgrades.

Body modification, whether medical or aesthetic, allows people to reclaim their bodies in ways that are deeply personal and profoundly meaningful. It is the ultimate marriage of biology and technology, humanity and innovation. It's not simply about fixing imperfections, but more rewriting the narrative of what's possible.

So whether you're a cyborg in the making or just someone who wants to pierce their eyebrow for fun, remember that modifying your body isn't merely an act of self-expression. It can be a testament to the resilience of the human spirit – and a reminder that, sometimes, being a little *extra* is exactly what we need.

BEAUTY IS PAIN?

As a species we've always been obsessed with aesthetics and are willing to put up with a bit of discomfort in the name of beauty or fashion. We could be talking about young men suffocating their genitals in a pair of skinny jeans or supermodels risking life and limb in twelve-inch heels. However, none of these come close to the impact that one particular 'fashion trend' had on generations of women: foot binding.

This extreme form of body modification was central to Chinese culture for almost a thousand years, causing untold deformities and chronic disabilities and sometimes even death. I must warn you, some of what I'm about to share is disturbing.

Picture a young girl, around four or five years old, living in imperial China. The planning for her marriage has already begun. In an attempt to make her as eligible as possible, the elders in the family begin by breaking the young girl's foot. Every one of the toes, except the big toe, is broken and forcibly rolled under the arch of the foot and wrapped tightly so they can't be straightened.

With feet resembling hooves, the girl is now forced to re-learn how to walk. In doing so, she endures unimaginable pain. If the breaking of the toes wasn't enough mangling, sometimes the elders would cut away pieces of the foot or mix glass shards into the binding to induce infections. The severe untreated infection would likely lead to necrosis and gangrene of the toes, causing them to fall off – all of this to ensure the smallest possible footprint and shoe size.

When the girl's foot healed in a contorted state, the breaking would happen again and again and again.

For almost ten centuries, generations of Chinese children endured this torturous form of body modification to conform to social expectations, as having intact, unbound feet was perceived as damaging for a girl's marriage prospects. The goal of the tiny 'lotus foot' adorned by an embroidered silken shoe was considered to be one of the most attractive qualities a prospective bride could possess. Naturally, the smaller the foot, the more erotically pleasing she was deemed to be – never mind the constant, life-long pain, the severely restricted mobility and the risk of further infection.

It wasn't until the twentieth century that the custom of foot binding began to fade, with the last known case recorded in 1957. Today foot binding is widely condemned and banished to the shameful archives of history; a deeply disturbing cultural tradition that was ruinous for generations of women.

Heels

Women wearing high heels may be less extreme than foot binding but it is another example of how society prioritises aesthetic appeal over physical comfort. Heels may elongate your legs, add height and confidence, but they can also be harmful to feet and musculoskeletal health.

When you're wearing 'flat' shoes, your body weight is distributed evenly. It means the shoe and your feet act as shock absorbers for your skeleton, cushioning the load. However, when women wear high heels, body weight is shifted forward on to the balls of the feet and the toes. This reduces shock absorption in your feet and results in greater discomfort. Heels of three inches or more can increase the load and pressure on your toes and balls of your feet by almost 80 per cent.

A high-heeled shoe also disproportionately increases the pressure in the big toe, known as the first metatarsal. This can increase the chances of bunion formation, or hallux valgus (where the big toe can splay outwards), not to mention things like corns or calluses.

While heels may look attractive to some, one thing that is decidedly less impressive is a Haglund's deformity. The chronic friction caused by wearing heels can result in a bump formation at the back of the heel that is often unsightly as well as painful.

It's not only the feet that are affected. Your spine normally has a nice S-shaped curve to it, designed to reduce the stress on each vertebra. As high heels push your body weight and centre of gravity forwards, your body adapts by flattening the lower spine as well as the hips and shoulders. Your natural body alignment is now further out of sync, resulting in abnormal loads on your spine and joints, which over time can lead to postural abnormalities, chronic pain and sciatica.

Habitual high-heel wearers might also suffer from knee pain. When wearing heels, the hips and shoulders pull back in an attempt to maintain some neutrality in your centre of gravity, which places more force on the ankles. High heels can also place a great amount of stress on the Achilles tendon at the back of the ankle, leading to future pain problems.

Of course, as with many medical issues, prevention is better than cure. So stop wearing heels – which I appreciate is unrealistic for many – or reduce the time you wear them. Let your feet have some time off just so the abnormal stresses are released temporarily. It won't just be your feet that are grateful but all the muscles and bones in your body that a pair of heels force out of position.

PLASTIC FANTASTIC

In recent decades, plastic surgery has grown significantly in popularity, and it encompasses various fields. Reconstructive surgery focuses on restoring appearance or function to patients with congenital defects, medical conditions or trauma, while cosmetic surgery aims to enhance physical appearance. The latter often attracts attention and controversy, highlighting the fact that beauty is often deeply subjective and culturally influenced.

A brief history of the boob job

Breast augmentation remains the most common and widely performed cosmetic surgery procedure and may be performed for aesthetic reasons or reconstructive purposes, particularly following cancer treatment. While breast implants have evolved significantly in the last few decades, the path to the modern boob job was one of serious trial and error, marked by disfiguring injections and a range of unsafe, experimental implant materials.

The German surgeon Vincenz Czerny performed the first documented breast reconstruction surgery using an implant in 1895. He transplanted a lipoma (a benign fatty tumour) from the patient's own body to plug a gap left by a cancerous tumour. Early in the twentieth century some unscrupulous practitioners were happily injecting paraffin wax into breast tissue to enlarge or reshape them. The results were instant and seemed decent enough, but came at a price. After a year or so, benign growths known as paraffinomas formed. These could be disfiguring, cause unbearable pain and in some cases led to breast amputation or even death.

During the Victorian era a variety of bizarre materials were implanted into breasts, from vegetable oils and goat's milk to sponges, cotton and even solid materials like spheres made from ivory. These often led to infections, rejections by the body and severe complications.

By the end of the Second World War, silicone injections had overtaken the 'paraffin boob job' in popularity; a trend fostered by Japanese sex workers, who injected silicone directly into their breast tissue to increase cup size.

The first time that structured silicone gel implants were used in breast surgery was 1962, by the American surgeons Thomas Cronin and Frank Gerow, on 29-year-old mother-of-six Timmie Jean Lindsay, from Houston, Texas. Timmie, believe it or not, had originally gone to see the plastic surgeons to get a tattoo removed and her ears fixed (which she believed stuck out too much). Nonetheless, Cronin and Gerow were able to convince her to be their human guinea pig for their experimental surgery. The silicone implants were far better than anything used before and influenced decades of future surgeries.

Breast reduction

While some patients need breast implants, others require breast reduction. For many, the decision is not about vanity; it's about reclaiming comfort, mobility and the ability to stand upright without their bra straps digging into their shoulders. For many women, it's less 'cosmetic surgery' and more 'Can I please have my life back?'.

Breasts are composed largely of fat and glandular tissue, and when they're on the larger side, they can each weigh 2–5kg. That's like strapping a pair of kettlebells to your chest every day. The added weight pulls the shoulders forward, straining the trapezius muscles, cervical spine and thoracic spine. This can lead to chronic back, neck and shoulder pain and large breasts can also compress the chest wall, restricting lung expansion and breathing.

Breast reduction surgery, or reduction mammoplasty, is a procedure that removes excess breast tissue, fat and skin. The benefits are immediate and far-reaching, and most women report dramatic reductions in back, neck and shoulder pain after surgery. Without the constant forward pull of heavy breasts, standing tall becomes an attainable reality rather than a pipe dream. Running, jumping or simply existing can be experienced without persistent discomfort.

And yet, despite its potential to significantly improve quality of life, obtaining breast reduction surgery can be an uphill struggle, often requiring the patient to repeatedly justify their pain and experience to healthcare providers. Add to that the complexities of healthcare systems like the NHS, where access to such procedures is rationed and often shrouded in red tape, and you've got a battle on your hands that rivals the sheer heft of the issue itself.

To qualify for surgery, patients are often required to demonstrate that their pain and discomfort have persisted despite non-surgical interventions like physiotherapy, painkillers or specialised bras. Many systems impose

This Is Vital Information

BMI thresholds for eligibility, ignoring the fact that losing weight doesn't magically shrink breasts made primarily of glandular tissue.

If you're struggling with large breasts and the system feels stacked against you, here's how to make your case.

- **Document everything**
    - Keep a symptom diary, noting back pain, shoulder grooves, bra-fitting difficulties and the impact on daily life.
    - Track expenses related to specialised bras, physiotherapy or pain management. It's not just about physical pain, but financial strain too.

- **Get medical backing**
    - Speak to your GP and ask for referrals to specialists like orthopaedic surgeons, physiotherapists or chronic pain clinics, who can provide supporting evidence for your case.
    - Request imaging (e.g., X-rays or MRIs) if possible, to document postural changes or spinal strain.

- **Highlight mental health impact**
    - Chronic pain isn't just physical; it can lead to anxiety, depression and body image issues. Be open about these challenges during consultations.

Is it worth it?

Humanity's obsession with bodies isn't new – just ask the Mayans, who filed their teeth into jaguar fangs, or the Victorians, who corseted their organs into oblivion. What's new is the scale: social media has turned self-loathing into a team sport. We've gone from tribal scarification to Facetune, trading ritual meaning for algorithmic validation. More teenagers are experiencing cyberbullying tied to appearance, proving that while technology evolves, our capacity for cruelty is still stuck in the Stone Age.

Body mod mayhem

That mole you contour into oblivion? The 'dad bod' you drown in Spanx? The universe doesn't care. It's too busy exploding stars and spinning galaxies to worry about your bingo wings. You're a sentient meat sack hurtling through space at 67,000mph on a rock that's 4.5 billion years old. The Milky Way doesn't notice if your brows are laminated. The universe isn't side-eyeing your muffin top.

Social media's beauty standards are just a flicker in humanity's endless, neurotic dance between belonging and individuality. In the grand vacuum of space, your 'flaws' are irrelevant. And maybe – just maybe – being cognisant of that is the route to freedom.

Confessions of a recovering meat puppet

For years, I was obsessed with my weight. Every fat person knows the feeling: the constant tugging at your shirt, the strategic angles in photos, the silent negotiations with mirrors before stepping out of the house. I spent an obscene amount of time trying to punish my body into submission; starving, sprinting, lifting, and googling cookie-cutter diet plans like they held the secrets of the universe.

Keto? Tried it. Paleo? Ate like a caveman for a bit. Vegan? Briefly converted, mostly out of desperation. Intermittent fasting? Yep, did it before it was cool and I just called that 'being too anxious to eat' in my twenties.

And for what? A six-pack? I've realised I'd much rather have a six-pack of soft bread rolls – warm, fluffy and satisfying. Because at some point, I realised two things:

- I love carbs
- My worth isn't defined by abs or arbitrary aesthetic ideals disguised as 'health'.

This Is Vital Information

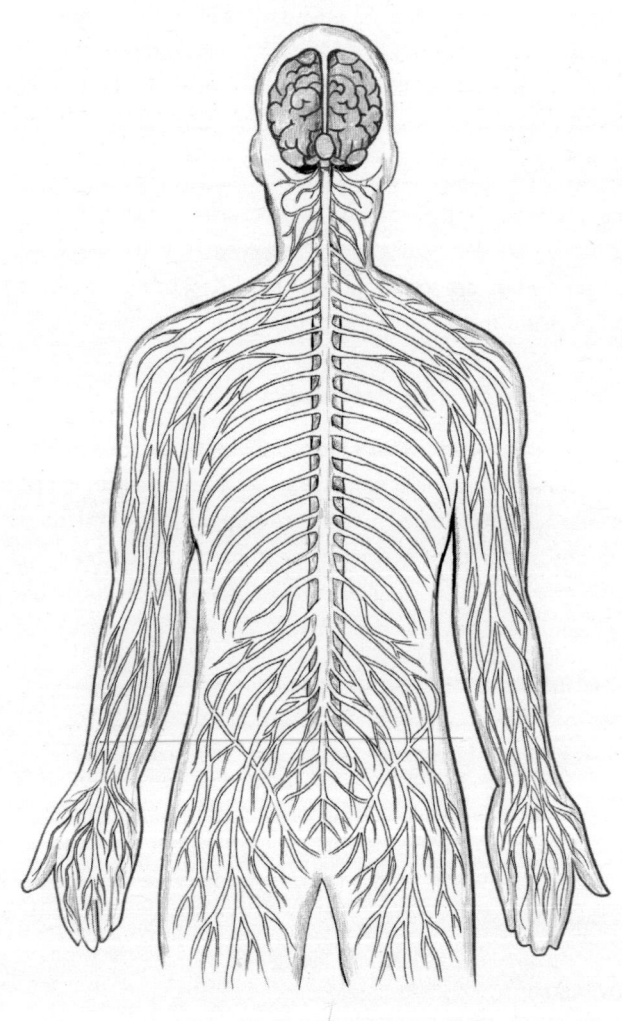

The central nervous system

Chapter 8

MESSING WITH THE MIND

MENTAL ILLNESS IS WIDE-RANGING AND COMPLEX, and part of a sprawling spectrum of conditions. I'm not a mental health expert so what follows is not a compendium of every mental health condition out there.

Instead, I would like to touch on a few that I have encountered personally and professionally, such as depression, anxiety and ADHD. They're the uninvited stragglers who show up everywhere: at work, at family dinners, in bed at 1am when you're trying to sleep. These conditions are pervasive, relatable, but also tragically misunderstood by everyone from your second cousin to the internet's worst advice-givers.

Disorders like schizophrenia, bipolar disorder, borderline personality disorder, obsessive-compulsive disorder (OCD) and more deserve their own dedicated discussions, ideally led by someone with clinical expertise and a good grasp of the latest research. These conditions often fly under the radar, cloaked in stigma and misunderstanding. Schizophrenia isn't just 'hearing voices'. Bipolar disorder isn't just 'mood swings'. They are deeply nuanced illnesses tied to complex neurochemical imbalances and structural brain changes. If you or someone you love suspects they might be dealing with any of these conditions, please, for the love of serotonin, dopamine and all the other neurotransmitters, see a professional. Self-diagnosis via TikTok will not save you.

I don't pretend I've cracked the code on mental health, nor does this chapter offer one-size-fits-all solutions. Instead, it's about pulling these conversations into the light, unpacking the science, and acknowledging that the human brain is an incredible, frustrating, beautifully messy machine that sometimes needs a bit of fine-tuning. And if we're being honest, don't we all?

The beauty of the brain

The brain sits at the top in more ways than one. Beyond simply having the highest altitude of any of your internal organs, it is also at the top of the organisational hierarchy. It is the executive organ, the overseer and commander of other body parts, like a general peering out of its vantage perch in its bony throne, the cranium.

Part of the brain's beauty lies in its complexity compared to other organs; a wildly elaborate and spider-like chain of electrical cells that is barely understood even by the brightest of scholars.

Your brain is the most advanced supercomputer in existence. It is a highly calibrated problem-solving machine. If you don't have a problem, fear not, your brain will find you one.

It is also a master of self-sabotage and prone to spurious malware infections and corrupted software: low mood, anxiety, stress, anger, frustration, questionable life choices, worry. The term mental health is relatively new, and attitudes towards it have changed for the better over recent years. It wasn't long ago that people were encouraged to 'snap out of it', and less than a century ago those deemed incurable were confined to asylums. In short, mental health concerns haven't always been something we've embraced as a society – which is why many still find it hard to ask for help when they're struggling.

Much of what we know about mental health, and how it goes wrong, is down to brain chemicals that have gone haywire. You might have a genetic predisposition that increases the chances of this happening but life stresses and various factors within and beyond your control also play a significant role.

WHAT IS MENTAL HEALTH?

Ask a psychologist, philosopher, psychiatrist and neuroscientist what mental health means and you'd probably get four very different answers. One might refer to clinical criteria or well-being scales measuring depression, distress or anxiety. Another might focus on patterns of behaviour or scan the brain for any abnormalities or underlying pathology.

How mental health is defined continues to vary both by era, field and person-to-person.

My own view of mental health is that the soft lump of fat in your skull exists in a state of balance; a homeostasis, if you will. Maintaining that balance requires flexibility and adaptability in response to shifting environments or life events. Sometimes we need help to do that, especially if our brains are 'wired' a little differently to others', and sometimes we need to work at it and give our minds a little care and attention.

Mental health awareness

The term mental health is everywhere in the modern world. We have mental health awareness days and weeks dotted throughout the year, not to mention the endless stream of self-help blogs, books, social media channels and more. Celebrities are also increasingly transparent about their own mental health struggles.

I'm all for raising awareness about mental health issues, but being aware of something isn't the same as truly understanding it. It's a bit like deep-fried food — everyone knows that a deep-fried piece of meat from your local takeaway is not exactly 'healthy' but people still eat it on occasion. With mental health, the challenge is even greater — and more nebulous and intangible than a greasy meal — making it harder to recognise when things are going wrong or what to do about it.

The human brain is also an obstinate beast, fixed in a certain way of thinking and it takes a lot more than saying something to change its belief systems. The brain is usually far more responsive to problems in the present moment than it is to abstract issues. You might not have any concerns about your home's central heating, but as soon as it stops working you're motivated to find out what's going on and get it fixed. This is natural; your brain prefers to focus on the now.

Similarly, you might not be experiencing any issues with your mental health but it is arguably more integral to your life than central heating. It also isn't a rare event. In the UK alone, 25 per cent of the population will experience a mental health problem every year – it's very much part of the human condition.

Hoof beats are horses, not zebras ...

When I was in my third year of medical school, just starting my clinical rotations, I heard one aphorism numerous times. Coined by Dr Theodore Woodward in the 1940s, it goes: 'If you hear hoof beats, think horses, not zebras.' Essentially, common things are just that. In the case of the unknown, the obvious is the most likely answer. Translated to medicine, a patient with a chronic cough is more likely to be suffering from a lung condition like asthma or COPD (chronic obstructive pulmonary disease) than a rare tropical disease (well, in the affluent suburbs of a London hospital at least).

People are far more familiar with physical problems as they're easier to spot than mental ones. If you see someone exuding bright red fluid from their backside, you know that isn't normal. The average person experiencing a mental health issue often doesn't have any obvious physical symptoms and what we portray to the world often belies the inner turmoil we are facing.

When things go wrong in the bone dome (aka the brain), I sometimes look at it as an adaptive strategy employed by the brain when it senses trouble. It's similar to how the body responds to inflammation in the gut lining, accelerating the digestive contractions to bring about a hasty chocolate flood, aka diarrhoea. The body is built for self-preservation, protection and survival and that flood of anxiety and stress is the legacy bestowed on us by prehistoric ancestors hardwired to flee from predators. A shot of adrenaline is undoubtedly handy if you're on the run from a woolly mammoth but not so useful when it's an overflowing inbox causing you stress.

Importantly, as I've found with many of my patients over the years, they're more likely to get better if they know why a certain problem exists rather than just looking at the symptoms. Granted, it is equally important to treat symptoms of low mood, stress and anxiety, but looking into the underlying causes is crucial too.

You can't be happy 100 per cent of the time. If you are, there is probably something very peculiar about you and I'd be interested in studying your brain. It is perfectly normal, however, to experience a full spectrum of negative emotions from time to time. More often than not, feeling 'off' can be put down to something very normal, just like those horse hooves. Occasionally, though, there's something more interesting at work, and we need to know when it's time to start looking for zebras. Unfortunately for our ancestors, they haven't always taken this approach.

Mental health through the ages

The treatment of mental illness is nothing new. Throughout history, various methods have been employed to treat mental health conditions – many of which now seem pretty barbaric.

In early civilisations, conditions of the mind were often attributed to supernatural causes such as possession by evil spirits or divine punishment. Sufferers were duly either cast out from a group or society, or were subjected to various unsavoury treatments, including exorcism, blood-letting or having holes drilled in their skulls to let out evil spirits, a process called trepanation. We still drill holes in skulls today but in a bid to let out 'evil' haematomas to equalise the pressure in the skull after a major bleed.

In Ancient Greece, the treatment and understanding of mental illness shifted away from the supernatural or religious sphere. The Greek physician Hippocrates – he of the Hippocratic Oath – saw mental illness as a physical disturbance, caused by an imbalance in the four 'humours' of the body: blood, yellow bile, black bile and phlegm. Treatment included blood-letting and daily purging, as well as dietary changes, rest and massages.

The Middle Ages saw a return to supernatural explanations for mental illness, from demonic possession to witchcraft, and the period saw a rise in witch-hunts and trials. Mental health illness may have played a role in the Salem witch trials in New England, when, in 1692, a group of young girls began exhibiting strange behaviour – convulsions, screaming and hallucinations. They in turn accused several women of witchcraft, which led to mass hysteria in the deeply religious Puritan community. Anxiety, post-traumatic stress disorder (PTSD), epilepsy, or a variety of undiagnosed mental health or neurological disorders may have led to the extreme behaviour, and one theory – still highly debated – postulates that ergot, a toxic rye fungus that contains alkaloids similar to LSD, may have caused the convulsions and delirium seen in the afflicted girls.

Whatever the causes, the persecutions and witch-hunts highlight how misunderstanding about mental health can often lead to stigma, scapegoating and ultimately violence. For centuries, people suffering from mental ill health were shunned, or seen as the responsibility and burden of their family, only to be hidden, locked up or abandoned altogether.

Institutions for the mentally ill did exist, particularly from the 1500s onwards, although many were primarily places of confinement and not of humane treatment. Many asylums merely repurposed prison-like institutions where 'undesirables' or those deemed disruptive to social order could be contained and kept out of public view.

The vast majority of asylums were staffed by unqualified individuals with little to no medical training and many abused their clientele. La Bicêtre, an asylum in Paris, was notorious for shackling patients to the walls in dark, cramped, unhygienic cells, forcing them to sleep standing up and live in their own excrement.

Patients were often subjected to grim conditions in the infamous London asylum, St Mary Bethlehem, nicknamed 'Bedlam'. In the seventeenth and eighteenth centuries, patients were put on display for the public to watch, like sideshow attractions, in exchange for one penny. Some were also sent out on to the streets to beg for money. Typical treatments for asylum patients included blood-letting, purging and cold baths, alongside an array of physical restraints that included straitjackets.

Open up and say 'Ah'

Attitudes to mental health, whether throughout history or today, stem from the outdated idea that physical health is tangible and therefore valid, while mental health is intangible and therefore suspect. It's why people feel more comfortable saying: 'I have the flu,' than 'I have anxiety.' No one questions the existence of viruses, but try explaining presynaptic terminals and neurotransmitters to your uncle over Christmas lunch.

The truth is, mental and physical health aren't separate categories; they're two sides of the same coin. Anxiety can spike your heart rate and blood pressure. Depression can mess with your sleep, appetite and immune system. Chronic stress can alter your gut microbiome and pave the way for a buffet of inflammatory diseases. The mind and body are a package deal, yet we persist in treating them as though one is real and the other is just a bad attitude.

Just because something is invisible it doesn't mean it's any less real or debilitating. You can't see a migraine, but no one doubts its existence when you're lying in a dark room cursing the light bulb that's suddenly your mortal enemy. You can't see diabetes either, but you'd never accuse someone of faking it because their pancreas decided to take early retirement. So why do we act like mental health issues are imaginary just because they don't come with a visible rash or a prescription for crutches?

This dismissal creates a dangerous level of shame in sufferers. People openly take antibiotics but feel the need to hide their antidepressants like they're stashing contraband. They might not go to work for a cold, but not for a bout of debilitating anxiety, even though both impair your ability to function.

The irony is almost poetic: the brain is the control centre for every single thing your body does, yet we treat its health as an afterthought. Mental health is physical health, full stop. The fact that you can't see serotonin levels doesn't make them less real. The fact that depression doesn't show up on an X-ray doesn't make it less crippling. And the fact that therapy and medication aren't visible badges of honour doesn't mean they're not life-saving tools. Talking to your therapist shouldn't feel like you're smuggling state secrets, yet here we are, treating therapy appointments like covert ops.

This stigma is absurd when you think about it. Imagine someone muttering softly: 'I've started seeing a personal trainer,' like it's a confession of deep shame. No, they announce it proudly, as though spending their Saturdays being yelled at to do burpees is a badge of honour. Therapy, on the other hand . . . somehow that's seen as a sign of weakness, as if trying to untangle the Gordian knot of your brain is less noble than building up biceps. We're fine with self-improvement when it's about abs, but mental health is apparently where we draw the line.

Similarly, taking medication for your mental health *should* be as unremarkable as taking ibuprofen for a headache. You're not weak or broken for needing a bit of pharmacological support. Your neurotransmitters and biology aren't staging a coup out of spite; it's chemistry, not character. If anything, it's a testament to your resilience and determination to feel better. You're not hiding a flaw but managing your health and that's something to respect, not ridicule.

The stigma around therapy and medication persists because we've conflated mental health struggles with personal failure. We've internalised the idea that we should be able to 'just deal with it' on our own. But let me tell you, nobody is out there bench-pressing their way out of depression or deadlifting their anxiety into submission.

Messing with the mind

If you need the scientific receipts, here they are: therapy and medication are evidence-based tools for managing mental health. Cognitive behavioural therapy (CBT) has been shown to rewire neural pathways, reducing symptoms of anxiety and depression. Medications like SSRIs (selective serotonin reuptake inhibitors) can help balance the neurotransmitters that contribute to the influence of mood and behaviour. These aren't magic pills or miracle cures, but effective strategies supported by decades of research.

Neuroscience even backs up the idea that seeking help is a smart move. The brain is a complex network of circuits that can get stuck in maladaptive patterns. Therapy helps you break those cycles, while medication provides the biochemical stability needed to make that change possible.

So how do we combat this stigma? By changing the narrative. Start by being open about your own mental health journey. Mention therapy in casual conversation, the same way you'd mention a workout class. If someone asks why you're taking medication, tell them it's because you value your health. Let's normalise the tools we use to heal, and the shame will start to dissipate.

And remember: there's no shame in being human. Life is hard, brains are complicated, and nobody gets through it unscathed. Seeing a therapist or taking medication isn't a sign that you're failing – it's a sign that you're trying. And in a world that often feels designed to grind us down, trying is the bravest thing you can do. So, hold your head high, pill bottle in hand, and take pride in your efforts to build a healthier, happier you. Because there's nothing embarrassing about wanting to be better.

The dark history of lobotomies

There was a time – just a few decades ago – when it was thought that people with severe mental health issues should have the two halves of their brain severed. Enter the lobotomy, one of the most brutal surgical procedures in recent memory, although it was once hailed as a miracle procedure.

Developed in 1935, this procedure was carried out for a wide range of conditions, from OCD to schizophrenia and learning disabilities. It was also administered to some patients as a means of controlling aggression (later embodied by the movie *A Clockwork Orange*). Although a very small minority of people saw an improvement in their symptoms, many were left in vegetative states or in a permanent stupor; unable to care for themselves, walk or even talk. So, how on earth did we think this was a good idea?

Faced with seemingly ineffective therapies for those afflicted with mental illness, Portuguese neurologist Egas Moniz developed the lobotomy, or the 'leucotomy' as he named it. The procedure involved drilling a pair of holes into the skull. This was followed by using a sharp instrument to cut into the brain tissue and then moving it from side to side to cut the connections between the frontal lobes and the remainder of the brain.

Based upon an anecdotal case series of twenty patients who experienced some improvements, Moniz declared his surgical technique to be a breakthrough. In America, these 'advances' piqued the interest of a young neurologist called Walter Freeman. In 1939, he performed the first lobotomy in the USA. Ten years later, in a bid to streamline the procedure, he devised the 'transorbital lobotomy' or 'ice pick lobotomy'. This involved hammering steel rods through the thin bone at the back of the eye socket and just above the eyelid. Freeman won widespread acclaim for his methods. His surgical work was covered by the *New York Times*, and became so popular that people across the country were lining up for their lobotomies.

One well-known patient was Rosemary Kennedy, sister of future US president John F. Kennedy. Growing up, Rosemary was known for being an outgoing, rebellious individual and a challenging daughter, according to her father. In 1941, he took Rosemary to see Walter Freeman. He diagnosed 'agitated depression' and conducted a corrective lobotomy immediately after diagnosis. A few days after the surgery it was evident that something was seriously wrong; Rosemary could no longer speak and her cognitive capabilities were reduced to that of a toddler. She was institutionalised by her father on the pretext that she was mentally unwell and it was only decades later that the truth behind the failed brain surgery was revealed.

The episode didn't put any dent in Freeman's reputation, however. Indeed, it encouraged him to reach more patients. The neurologist took to the road and toured health institutions around the country in his van, which was known as the 'Lobotomobile'. At his peak, Freeman was conducting twenty-five lobotomies in a single day for conditions as basic as headaches. Sometimes, he would perform the procedure on patients as young as four years old.

Over the next four decades, Freeman performed more than 3,500 lobotomies despite no formal surgical training or research into his methods. Eventually, with a growing understanding of neuroscience and neurology and the adverse effects of the lobotomy, the procedure was banned in several countries. As the poor results became increasingly apparent, it was also discovered that Freeman had a mortality rate of 15 per cent – meaning fifteen out of every one hundred patients died as a result of the procedure. Not great odds for any procedure.

In today's world, any surgeon using an operating technique with a mortality rate of 15 per cent and no guarantee of 'cure' would be behind bars. It's worth noting that Freeman, though he very quickly lost the respect of his peers, never actually ended up in court nor was he ever sued for medical malpractice or negligence (even though many a time he took photos while shoving an ice pick halfway into someone's fatty lump of head flesh).

The tale of the Ice Pick Man nears its end in 1967. He received a visit from Helen Mortensen, one of his first patients who received a transorbital lobotomy. Freeman performed a second and subsequently third lobotomy on her as she suffered relapse after relapse of her psychiatric symptoms.

The third time was no lucky charm in this case as he ended up puncturing a blood vessel in her brain, which led to her death a few days later. The hospital where Freeman conducted his 'surgery' revoked his ability to practise on its premises. This would be the last lobotomy of his career. In 1972 he died from cancer at the age of seventy-six, with his shadow still casting a deep darkness over the field of both neurosurgery and psychiatry.

HOW THE BRAIN WORKS

In order to understand what can go 'wrong' in the brain, we need to know what happens when it's going 'right'. If you want to be a surgeon and comprehend the disease process of bowel conditions, you need to have a grip of anatomical basics that go all the way to the top. Frankly, the last thing you want to hear from your surgeon is 'Hey, what's that?' I could continue to explain all sorts of weird and wonderful stories of neuroscience but without the basics in place I might as well spend the next few pages spelling out fart noises.

Inner workings of the brain

Like everything in your body, the brain is comprised of cells. In the case of the stuff that makes up our grey matter, these cells are bestowed the title of neurons. Collectively, they look like a hybrid tree-spider organism. They can also be found across your entire nervous system: your spinal cord and all the nerves that permeate every crevice of your body. In fact, it could be said that you are essentially a walking nervous system tightly wrapped in a meat cage.

In addition to the neurons, you have specialised support cells known as glial cells, which grease the wheels of the neurons. Think of them as the pit-stop crew or the scrub nurse to the neuron's surgeon – existing to support, protect and assist. Each cell has a central part called the cell body. Extending from the cell body are tree-branch-like dendrites, which help receive signals from other neurons. Shooting off the main cell body is a big thick tree-trunk appendage called an axon. These axons are bundled together to form nerves and serve as the electrical hardware of the body.

The brain itself contains around 86 billion neurons and 100 trillion connections. Essentially, these facilitate you taking a dump or making your pasta dinner. They're also involved in your panic attack or forgetting to set your alarm clock making you late for work.

I'm not going to bore you with the intricacies of electrical activity and the physics of membrane potentials. Because I despised this stuff at medical school and still do. (And also, in all honesty, it has very little relevance to what you need to know over the next few pages; it's the neuroscience equivalent of learning differential equations in maths.) To put it simply: the surfaces of all these cells are highly electrically active, like microscopic batteries with a small voltage across them. This seemingly negligible amount of electrical charge is the crux of life and everything you do. What's more, the charge can spread out, away from one point, and travel along the length of the neuron, just like ripples in a pond. We're not talking about random bursts of activity but ripples of energy that can be intentionally directed to specific locations. They can be amplified, hastened and modulated in a number of ways and used to encode complex information like a biological version of Morse code.

At this very moment, the billions of neurons in your brain are bursting with electrical activity to visualise, process and understand the words you're reading on this page. This happens trillions of times every second of every day and is the source of every movement, thought, action or sensory experience you've ever had. It's not just a mound of grease and fat stored in bone, but it's pivotal in all that is good and, unfortunately, a lot of what is bad too.

Most neurons, or 'brain cells', aren't directly connected but signal to each other via the release of neurotransmitters or chemicals that travel in the small gap between them. Think of neurotransmitters as beacons between a cascade of falling items. They take the message from one neuron and pass on the Mexican wave of electrical activity to the next.

It's also important to understand that neurons don't just form long daisy chains with other neurons. They tangle with each other, form loops, side branches, weird junctions and all sorts of fanciful and bizarre arrangements. If you thought your headphone wires becoming tangled was bad, that is nothing compared to the biological twister that is the human brain. Ultimately, the neurons' aim is to maintain the connections that allow us to function from one millisecond to the next throughout the course of our lives.

Of course, the brain is more than just a power generator pumping out pulses of energy in complicated ways. It can also inform the character of each pulse by triggering the release of neurotransmitters such as dopamine, serotonin and oxytocin. These function like hormones in the bloodstream and can have different effects depending on how they are deployed and in what concentration. In shaping the way we think and behave, the brain also forms our entry point for understanding mental health.

Brain versus the mind

The first time I held a human brain it was somewhat heavier than the 1.3kg or so that I expected. Perhaps I should have felt enlightened or maybe even humbled? In reality, my own brain was having to contest with the idea of holding another brain. All I could think about was the sheer weight of the thing.

The existential right hook came a few moments later.

You can't just pick up a normal human brain that hasn't been treated with preservative chemicals. It's far too fragile. The preservation fluid allows it to undergo a chemical hardening process so that the consistency of it can settle.

As I looked at the brain again, wondering about the possibilities of the neurons contained within going haywire across this person's life, it was hard to not be overwhelmed by the realisation that this mass of tissue in

Messing with the mind

my hands was an entire life not too long ago. A person's dreams, hopes, fears and insecurities were catalogued inside; every book, movie or piece of music they'd enjoyed, and potentially deep-rooted mental health issues and despair as well.

I positioned the specimen on the metallic surface of the dissecting room table, just like in Andreas Vesalius's series of books on human anatomy, *De humani corporis fabrica libri septem* (*On the Fabric of the Human Body*), and stared down. In front of me was one of the greatest mysteries of the world. The squishy organ that created and maintained the autonomous rhythm of life. After carefully inspecting every crevice and crenulation, and delineating the vascular anatomy as it tangled around the soft tissue, I finally stepped away and moved on to the next organ. In those twenty minutes, I had one person's everything – from cognition to cosmos – in my grasp.

Given the brain is arguably the most advanced piece of technology we are ever likely to come across (at least in our lifetime), I find it useful to think about it as expensive hardware and our mind, mental health and personality as the software. For a well-functioning computer devoid of glitches, both need to be regularly maintained. For example, lack of sleep can result in a gradual corrosion of your hardware (you will have increased levels of cortisol and other stress hormones and you miss out of the cerebrospinal fluid brain wash), which can then impact the software, making you fatigued, irritable and low in mood.

It is perfectly reasonable to assume that, just like a computer, your software, hardware, RAM and processing speed can be 'tweaked' by medication, lifestyle change, social factors and more.

Now that we've established that your brain and body and by extension life itself are a series of chemical reactions and messages, it's also reasonable to think that these chemical messages can be 'rewired', or hijacked, via external cues or chemicals that tell your brain to do something else entirely.

Extrapolating this idea of chemicals causing disturbances in the brain, you might then subscribe to the 'chemical imbalance' theory of depression.

This Is Vital Information

You wouldn't be alone because the majority of people think this. You'd also be incorrect.

This idea is ingrained in pop psychology and even has a plethora of research behind it. I was even taught this in medical school, so it's easy to see how we might be fooled.

The chemical that is off balance in this theory of depression is serotonin, a neurotransmitter that provides 'feel-good' effects. Serotonin is somewhat of a jack of all trades; it plays a part in your sex drive, appetite, alertness, body temperature regulation and much more. It seems reasonable to infer that having low levels of serotonin could lead to low mood or mental illness, making it important to increase its levels in the fight against depression.

However, psychiatrists and academics have since realised the 'chemical imbalance' theory doesn't explain the complexities of depression and it has since ended up in the academic wastebin. The problem is they forgot to inform the public.

Pharmaceutical companies have *some* (that's me being generous) role to play in the extended shelf life of this worn-out theory. Drug companies who create and sell antidepressants, like selective serotonin reuptake inhibitors (SSRIs), continue to send out messages like 'this may help to correct this imbalance by increasing the brain's own supply of serotonin'. This isn't to say that SSRIs don't work; it's more that they probably aren't as effective as we would like them to be but they are still more effective than placebos or doing nothing at all.

Academics in mental health, in fact, have known for a number of years that the role of serotonin deficiency and depression has been overstated and that something as complex as depression cannot be reliant on one chemical.

One large literature review published in 2022, which questioned the serotonin theory of depression, garnered significant media attention and began sounding the death knell for the chemical imbalance theory, at least in its current form. The review suggested that there was no convincing evidence that a reduced serotonin level is a causative factor in, or is even associated with, depression. As to what does cause depression, the answer is far from simple, sending psychiatric researchers back to the drawing board in their quest to understand the condition.

From tuberculosis to serotonin

As unlikely as it may sound, the whole serotonin debate has its roots in the treatment of tuberculosis in the 1950s.

Iproniazid was originally created to target mycobacterium tuberculosis in the lung, but doctors noticed that patients taking the drug seemed more cheerful and energetic. Puzzled by this, researchers investigated further and discovered that iproniazid increased the levels of certain chemicals, particularly serotonin. This led to the decades-long notion that depression was linked to deficiencies in certain chemicals, most notably serotonin. This influenced the development of drugs for depression and even today, when patients are prescribed SSRIs, the explanation they are given is the serotonin hypothesis.

While we know that depression isn't caused solely by a deficiency in serotonin, clinical trials show that, while responses vary, SSRIs do alleviate symptoms of depression but we are yet to fully understand *how* they work. SSRIs affect other chemicals in the brain alongside serotonin and this may go some way to explain their effectiveness.

We now also have evidence that a wide range of genes – i.e., segments of your DNA – are linked to depression. Having these genes doesn't mean you're destined to be depressed as these genes also need certain biological or environmental conditions to be activated.

There is also good evidence that chronic inflammation raises the risk of depression as it can hinder the body's ability to repair and heal. Inflammation can cause a deterioration of synaptic connections in neural tissue, which can contribute to mood disorders. We have evidence of this connection in patients who suffer with chronic inflammatory conditions like rheumatoid arthritis or lupus, and who have notably higher levels of depression. However, this could be a 'chicken and egg' situation, where depression somehow is contributing towards inflammation in the first place.

EVERYTHING YOU KNOW ABOUT ADHD IS WRONG

If you've stepped foot in the digital world, you'll have been inundated by a digital cacophony of videos about ADHD (attention deficit hyperactivity disorder). It's a condition that has been the subject of a huge amount of stigma, scrutiny and debate, with some people even questioning its very existence.

ADHD is complex and is more than the stereotype of a hyperactive person or someone with a short attention span. It is one of the most poorly understood brain conditions – in fact, it's likely that everything you know about ADHD is wrong. So before we go any further, let's talk about what ADHD actually is.

ADHD is classified, certainly by the NHS, as a neurodevelopmental condition that arises from differences in how the brain develops and functions, which in turn affects behaviour. Having ADHD doesn't automatically lead to poor mental health, but symptoms can trigger or exacerbate mental health issues or coexist alongside other conditions.

ADHD is a disorder of the brain evidenced by structural differences on brain scans and imaging studies of people with ADHD. MRI studies show that people with ADHD have smaller amygdalae (the part of the brain responsible for keeping emotions in check) and hippocampi (two little seahorses in the brain taking care of memory and learning) than their peers.

As a result, someone with ADHD can be termed as 'neurodivergent' in that the variations in their brain are natural and not 'neurotypical' – other neurodivergent conditions include autism, Tourette syndrome and dyslexia.

Messing with the mind

Beyond an anatomical or structural difference, there are also chemical alterations in the ADHD brain such as deficiencies in various neurotransmitters like dopamine. These have direct effects on the brain reward pathways, which can affect motivation, drive, attention, emotional regulation, communication and more.

Symptoms of ADHD can manifest in myriad ways. These include:

- Carelessness or lack of attention to detail
- Poor organisational skills and inability to focus and prioritise
- Forgetfulness and continually losing things
- Restlessness and often interrupting conversations
- Mood swings and risky behaviour.

The problem is a lot of these symptoms are common in people without ADHD, just to a lesser extent (but not always). Who doesn't have trouble multitasking or following through with a particularly boring admin task? And who isn't fighting the urge to impulse-scroll social media from 2 to 4pm?

I spoke to a celebrity couple on my podcast who had three neurodivergent children, all of whom had ADHD, and the one line that really struck me in the conversation was this: 'If you meet a child with ADHD, you've met *one* child with ADHD.'

ADHD is a label, but this belies its nuances and subtypes, which offer unique symptoms. Just as people have diverse traits, so does ADHD manifest differently in individuals and some of these unique symptoms are overlooked and misdiagnosed.

TikTok and social media might make you think all you have to do is watch a few videos with relatable aspects and make a self-diagnosis. This is not the case. ADHD has lots of coexisting conditions, meaning that someone with ADHD has a higher risk of issues like depression, anxiety, dyslexia and so on.

Sometimes it is difficult to unpick whether they are two separate conditions that require separate treatment or whether the coexisting one is secondary to ADHD. ADHD symptoms can also be mirrored by other medical conditions and mental health issues. The symptoms attributed to ADHD can often be caused by a host of other issues, including anxiety, sleep problems, bipolar and other mood disorders, thyroid problems, iron deficiency, hormonal changes, allergies, autism . . . I could go on.

There's also a belief that ADHD sufferers can control their symptoms, that they are not trying hard enough to be 'normal'. In reality, those with ADHD often have to spend greater mental energy to complete tasks than their neurotypical counterparts, meaning they're already trying harder.

Diagnosing ADHD

Another challenge with ADHD is that it's often an invisible condition and many people – especially girls and women – suppress or hide their symptoms. Unlike the more obvious hyperactive, disruptive behaviours seen in some boys, girls with ADHD can appear quieter or more daydreamy, meaning their condition is frequently overlooked or misdiagnosed.

The general trend, however, is that more people are being diagnosed with ADHD. The number has risen by about 160 per cent between 1997 and 2016, and the trend is continuing. In part this is due to an increased awareness of ADHD and the stigma around it slowly eroding. Social media has played a big part in spreading this awareness and destigmatising the condition, so that's a big plus. But the information shared on these platforms isn't always accurate.

A study from the University of British Columbia and the University of Toronto found that 52 per cent of the 100 most-watched ADHD videos on TikTok were misleading. That's concerning, given that the clips in the study had an average of 3 million views each. Only 21 per cent of the top 100 videos were found to have scientifically correct information about ADHD and only 11 per cent were uploaded by healthcare professionals.

'Most of these misleading videos oversimplified ADHD, recommended incorrect treatments or wrongly attributed symptoms of other psychiatric disorders as being a symptom of ADHD,' the study's authors said. Not ideal.

As a result, many of these videos could be spreading misinformation about mental health, reinforcing oversimplified stereotypes, overlooking coexisting conditions like anxiety and depression, and fuelling a concerning trend for self-diagnosis that risks minimising the real challenges people face.

It's great that people are talking about ADHD online, but you can't trust everything you read (or watch) on the internet. So take the information you learn from there with a pinch of salt, do plenty of your own due diligence, and if you can, try to speak to a healthcare professional before drawing any conclusions.

Perfectly imperfect

I am very uncomfortable with imperfection. As a surgeon, the sense of responsibility for other people and making life and death decisions drives this sense of discomfort around fallibility.

I've been operating for a number of years, but progress doesn't just reach a plateau. Being a doctor and especially a surgeon is about constantly refining your craft and seeking technical improvements, even if it's by 0.1 per cent; that could make a critical difference to a patient.

But no matter how good you are and how low your complication rates, the inescapable fact is that all surgeons have to deal with unintended problems or occurrences during surgery.

My old boss once told me: 'If a surgeon says they've had no complications it means one of two things – they are a liar or they don't operate enough. It's statistics.'

I learned this the hard way when performing a routine appendectomy earlier in my career. This particular morning, as I entered a young man's abdomen, I found it completely blackened, covered in pus and necrotic (essentially dead) tissue. The abdomen was hostile – surgical slang for a challenging or dangerous environment – and there was a great deal of inflammation, making everything bleed just at the touch and generally buggering up the ease of the operation.

At this point in my training, I had more than 100 appendix operations under my belt and felt pretty confident I could handle anything that came my way.

An hour and a half into the operation, I'd managed to clear up most of the infection, free the appendix, and was getting ready to remove it when I decided to call my boss to confirm I'd not missed anything obvious. He popped in, confirmed everything looked good and that he was happy, gave me a nod and left the operating room.

Two weeks later I was on call and I saw a familiar-sounding patient name in A&E. It was the patient whose appendix I'd removed. His CT scan showed he had a small infection around the region where the appendix had been removed. My first complication.

I informed my boss and he seemed nonchalant. 'It was inevitable. The initial infection and inflammation was so bad . . . this was bound to happen . . . nothing you could have done to prevent this.'

Although the patient didn't require a second operation, just a course of antibiotics for a week to treat this infection, I took this as a personal failure, despite what my boss said. I had failed my patient and myself.

This perception of personal failure lingered with me to the point where over the next few weeks I felt waves of anxiety every time I performed surgery with my bosses. It got to the point where I fervently hoped I wouldn't be needed or called upon to operate.

My mental turmoil was a combination of guilt, wanting to hide, feeling unworthy of my profession, and I even questioned my career choice. I ruminated myself into a negative cycle where I admonished myself for not being good enough and became more withdrawn from my peers. It was only through help from my mentor that I began to reframe my internal narrative and march through the abyss I was dragging myself into.

This was an extreme scenario but I'd be lying if I said clinicians and healthcare professionals didn't suffer from high levels of anxiety on a frequent basis. In fact, it would be strange if we didn't – we are, after all, expected to make life-changing decisions and prescribe potent and sometimes lethal drugs to patients, some of whom are precipitously close to death's door. We also make mistakes, and sometimes the result of these mistakes causes grievous harm and, in the worst case, death.

But it might reassure you to know that I and many people in medicine genuinely worry about the people we care for. This is anxiety driven by a sense of purpose, by a concern that walks a tightrope between blind panic (on occasion) and reckless conviction, settling over time into an equilibrium of part vigilance and part confidence.

When I do my ward rounds and obsessively stare at my patient's physiological parameters on the iPad screen, the human body (usually) does a fairly good job at maintaining core body temperature, blood pressure, electrolyte levels and other key variables to sustain life. However, if one parameter runs amok and prompt action is not taken, then the patient can fall into a serious condition.

Just like the body's biological parameters, anxiety is another facet of the human condition that can vary considerably on a day-to-day basis. Too much and it can be overpowering and paralysing.

What people get wrong about anxiety is that they see it as a psychological experience, but it is also a physical one. Anxiety can be driven by fear, but it differs in that fear is linked to a specific cause, whereas anxiety can exist in and of itself.

This Is Vital Information

Anxiety can manifest in myriad ways and many of these end up aggravating the situation. There are intricate paths that connect the skin and the brain, for example. During end-of-year exams at medical school, one of my housemates would frequently have an acne flare-up while he buried himself under a mountain of medical textbooks and emotional stress.

During periods of stress your brain releases corticotropin-releasing hormone (CRH), which stimulates the pituitary gland inside your brain box, to secrete adrenocorticotropic hormone (ACTH), which finally makes its way to the adrenal glands to encourage the production of cortisol and worsen acne, increasing oil (sebum) production and skin inflammation. It's no surprise that stress can worsen many inflammatory skin conditions like psoriasis and eczema.

Anxiety can mildly tickle your stomach and give rise to 'butterflies', or spill over into nausea if driven by extreme levels of anxiety before an exam or job interview. Beyond this, it can give rise to the dreaded 'anxiety poop', where the flood of stress chemicals mess with the gentle balance of your intestines and cause a great flood of chocolate liquid as your intestinal motility is sped up. Anxiety can trigger palpitations, breathlessness, a fast heart rate, sometimes even boiling over to the feeling of impending doom and imminent death.

Anxiety is an inescapable part of life and, in fact, even a superpower in small doses, but it can also go rogue and become an unwelcome guest in our lives.

Wrestling with stress

Stress is the parasite of modern existence. It's the tax we pay for being creatures with oversized brains and 24/7 Wi-Fi access, and, unlike your to-do list (which may be the source of your woes), stress can't be deferred. It's here, it's relentless, and it's always looking for ways to mess you up.

But don't despair, stress isn't the enemy. At least, not entirely. It's a survival mechanism designed by evolution to keep you alive. Unfortunately, evolution didn't anticipate your boss's cryptic Slack messages or the existential dread of climate change. So here we are, armed with fight-or-flight instincts that are a bit much for dealing with an empty milk carton. Let's break down stress, how it works, and what you can do to manage it without spiralling into a doom-scroll abyss.

Step 1: Know thy enemy (the physiology of stress)

Stress begins in the hypothalamus, a little almond-shaped tyrant in your brain. When it senses danger, whether it's an actual tiger or just a co-worker who ends every email with 'per my last', it hits the panic button, activating your sympathetic nervous system. This sets off the HPA (hypothalamic–pituitary–adrenal) axis, your body's stress command centre.

What happens next is pure chaos. Cortisol and adrenaline are released, raising your heart rate and blood pressure; your amygdala, the emotional drama queen of the brain, goes into overdrive; and meanwhile, your prefrontal cortex (the rational part) takes a backseat, leaving you prone to impulsive decisions like rage-quitting your job or buying an air fryer you don't need.

This cascade is helpful if you're running from a predator, but less so when you're running late for the bus.

Step 2: Start with your breath (your built-in brake system)

Your breath is the only part of your autonomic nervous system you can control at will, making it your stress-response cheat code. Deep breathing activates the parasympathetic nervous system, which is essentially your body's 'chill out' button. Deep, slow breaths signal to your vagus nerve (our old friend) to calm things down. Heart rate slows, blood pressure drops, and cortisol takes a hike.

Practical tip: Your exhale is key. Longer exhales stimulate relaxation. You can also try box breathing:

inhale for four seconds, hold for four, exhale for four, hold for four. Repeat.

Step 3: Move your body (but don't overthink it)

Stress lives in your muscles. Literally. When your body gears up for action but never gets to use that adrenaline (because no one actually sprints away from work emails), it has nowhere to go. Movement releases that tension and triggers endorphins, your body's natural opioids.

How it works:

- Exercise lowers cortisol levels and increases brain-derived neurotrophic factor (BDNF), a protein that helps your brain grow new neurons and recover from stress damage.

- Physical activity also increases serotonin and dopamine levels, giving you an instant mood boost.

What to do:

- Go for a brisk walk. This doesn't have to be a soul-searching trek. Just ten to twenty minutes around the local park will do.

- Dance like an idiot. Your brain doesn't care if you look ridiculous; it just wants you to move.

Step 4: Get a grip on your mind (before it spirals)

Your brain loves a good catastrophe. It's a survival trait gone rogue, constantly scanning for threats and imagining worst-case scenarios. The trick here is learning to stop this cycle without slapping your inner monologue in the face.

How it works:

- Practices like mindfulness and cognitive reframing engage the prefrontal cortex, calming the amygdala and breaking the loop of stress-induced overthinking.

Practical tips:

- **Name it to tame it:** Label your stress (e.g., this is anxiety about that deadline). This simple act reduces emotional intensity, a phenomenon backed by fMRI studies.

- **Flip the script:** Instead of thinking: 'I'm so overwhelmed,' try 'This is hard, but I've handled hard things before.' It sounds cheesy, but it works.

Step 5: Sleep like it's your job

Stress messes with sleep, and lack of sleep makes stress worse. It's the cruellest feedback loop. Sleep is when your brain cleans the house, flushing out stress by-products and resetting your nervous system. Without it, you're basically trying to fight a dragon with a toothpick.

How to hack it:

- Set a bedtime. Then stick to it.

- Limit your caffeine intake after midday – it can hang around in your system for up to ten hours.

- Try a wind-down ritual: dim the lights, read something boring, and avoid TikTok rabbit holes.

Stress isn't something you beat once and for all. The goal isn't to eliminate it entirely but to live alongside it without letting it ruin your life. And when all else fails, remember: you're just a flawed, glorious bag of neurons doing your best. That's enough.

This Is Vital Information

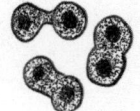 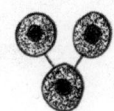 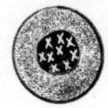 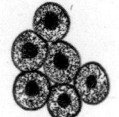

Normal, healthy cells

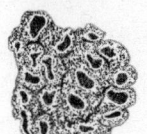 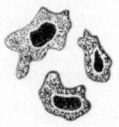 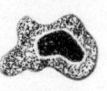 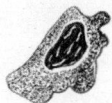 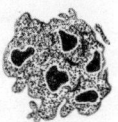

Cancerous cells

Chapter 9

THE BIG C

ALTHOUGH MY JOB INVOLVES HEALING and fixing things and cutting out the bad, sometimes I feel like the Grim Reaper. I bestow the worst possible news to some patients.

During a busy week of on-call shifts, just as I was about to take my lunch break, I checked the patient waiting room and spotted an elderly gentleman who was the exact shade of Homer Simpson. A knot formed in my stomach and erased my appetite. Stuffing my sandwich back into my bag, I knew I had to see him immediately and I feared the worst as I called his name.

He sat down in the examination room and was accompanied by his wife, who also seemed to have a tinge of jaundice about her and a yellowing of the whites of her eyes. This was going from awful to devastating.

A thorough history revealed the gentleman had experienced 'indigestion-like' pain for a few months (epigastric pain), that his trousers had become looser (unintentional weight loss) and his skin was increasingly yellow (jaundice). Given his advanced age, the first thing in my mind was pancreatic cancer.

I organised some blood tests for him and an urgent CT scan. Although his wife wasn't a patient, I hesitated for a second in case I was being too nosy but asked if she or anyone else had noticed her jaundice. She told me she was waiting for a doctor's appointment but was also experiencing some similar symptoms to her husband. I asked if she wouldn't mind if I asked her some more detailed questions and examined her.

Three hours later, and after obsessively refreshing the screen waiting for the two CT reports for the married couple, the news was in. My fears were confirmed. The elderly gentleman had a large pancreatic cancer compressing his bile ducts and blocking the flow of bile into his intestines, which explained his jaundice. Thankfully his wife just had gallstones, which was still serious but crucially *not* cancer. The universe wasn't feeling quite so cruel that day.

I've lost count of the number of times I've broken the news of cancer to people. In doing so, I've witnessed and felt the full gamut of emotions. As a nervous and shy first-year doctor, I bumbled through an awful skin cancer diagnosis to a 49-year-old maths teacher, while as a seasoned surgical doctor I had to tell a 35-year-old mother of four that she had bowel cancer and watched her collapse on me as she processed the weight of the news. I've seen it all and it's never easy.

Perhaps even more surprisingly, I've also seen dozens of patients who, in the face of a cancer diagnosis, simply shrug and mumble a variation of the phrase 'It is what it is. So what now?'

The elderly gentleman with pancreatic cancer was in the latter category. His response to his diagnosis – 'Oh right. That's not good then is it?' – was in contention for understatement of the year. His cancer was inoperable and he would likely be dead within a few months, if not weeks. Many patients ask 'how long?' when they receive the worst news in the world. But he didn't. He held his wife's hands and kissed her on the cheek. All I could utter at that moment was 'I'm sorry, sir'.

CANCER: THE WORD THAT STOPS CONVERSATIONS (AND, OCCASIONALLY, PEOPLE)

There are words in the English language that carry enough weight to stop a conversation mid-sentence. Some words make people blush (*sex*), some make them cringe (*moist*), but no word has quite the silence-inducing, existential dread-triggering power as *cancer*.

You could be mid-dinner party, discussing something utterly mundane – whether tomatoes belong in the fridge, or is pineapple a war crime on pizza – when someone utters the word. Suddenly, cutlery clatters, throats are cleared, someone nervously changes the subject to *literally anything else*, and suddenly it's as if we're all collectively trying not to summon Voldemort.

And yet, when I told that elderly patient that he had cancer, he just nodded, as if he'd been informed that his soup was slightly under-seasoned, while the room around him bristled with unspoken tension. He had, I imagine, seen enough of life's absurdity to know that fear of a word changes nothing about the reality of it.

But the unfortunate reality of life is that one in two of us will get cancer in our lifetimes. That's not a vague warning; that's the statistical equivalent of a coin toss. Half of us will face the Big C head-on, and the other half will love someone who does. This isn't some distant, improbable spectre.

Yet we still treat it like a linguistic landmine, as though avoiding the word will somehow stop cells from stabbing us in the back. But cancer doesn't care about our avoidance. It doesn't whisper. It invades, hijacks, mutates and multiplies like an exceptionally aggressive corporate takeover happening inside your own body. And still we struggle to say it out loud.

Cancer is not a mysterious, otherworldly force. It's biology with a tragic sense of humour. Cells are supposed to die, and when they don't, we get cancer. It's less a curse and more a clerical error in cellular mortality.

So, if half of us are going to deal with it anyway, isn't it time we stopped treating cancer like a dark secret and started accepting it for the public health crisis that it is? Instead of whispering, we should be talking loudly and frequently. Because knowledge, early detection and research save lives. Avoidance does not.

This Is Vital Information

So, let's see what all the fuss is about. Because pretending cancer doesn't exist has never stopped anyone from getting it.

Cancer 101

Given how common cancer is, it's surprising how many people don't really know what it is. Beyond being a 'bad thing', what actually is cancer?

When you ask someone to define cancer, they might offer vague descriptions: 'bad cells', 'something about tumours', or 'the thing that happens when you eat microwave food from plastic containers'.

So let's shed some light here: cancer is a biological glitch; a programming error. Your body is made up of trillions of cells, all of which follow strict rules: grow, function, divide when necessary, then die like a responsible adult when their time is up. This organised chaos is controlled by DNA, which acts as the instruction manual. Cancer occurs when this manual gets corrupted like a bad software update, but instead of your phone glitching, your cells forget how to die.

Normal cells divide only when needed; cancer cells divide whenever they damn well please. Normal cells respect boundaries; cancer cells spread and invade other tissues like a biological gentrification project. Normal cells know when to self-destruct (apoptosis); cancer cells develop god complexes and refuse to die.

This insubordination starts when mutations occur in key genes that regulate cell growth. The biggest offenders are oncogenes and tumour suppressor genes. Oncogenes are the accelerators of cell division. When mutated, they get jammed in the 'pedal to the metal' position, making cells divide uncontrollably. Tumour suppressor genes, meanwhile, are the brakes, designed to stop runaway growth. If these get damaged, the cell is left barrelling forward with no way to stop, like a horrible traffic accident happening inside your body, except the cars (cells) don't crash – they just keep multiplying until they clog up entire organs.

The Big C

Cancer doesn't just happen. It's the result of accumulated damage over time, and the culprits can vary. Here's a non-exhaustive, terrifyingly broad list of what can cause cancer:

- **Carcinogens:** Chemicals, radiation, smoking, UV exposure, the usual suspects
- **Genetic predisposition:** Some people, thanks to their ancestry, are born with mutations that make cancer more likely (thanks, Dad)
- **Viral infections:** HPV, hepatitis B/C and Epstein–Barr virus can all hack your DNA like a rogue programmer
- **Chronic inflammation:** Prolonged inflammation stresses your cells, leading to more mutations. Think of it as microscopic road rage inside your tissues.

The longer you live, the more cellular mistakes you accumulate, which is why cancer is more common as we age; your DNA has simply been through too many rounds of proofreading errors.

Not all cancers are created equal, and some are more aggressive than others. But in general, what makes cancer so uniquely terrifying is its ability to:

- **Evade the immune system:** Your immune system is usually great at identifying rogue cells and eliminating them. But cancer develops cloaking mechanisms, making it invisible to the body's defence forces.
- **Angiogenesis (building its own blood supply):** Cancer tricks your body into growing blood vessels to feed itself, like a parasite demanding table service.
- **Metastasis (spreading to other organs):** The deadliest feature of cancer is its ability to break off and travel to distant parts of the body. What started in the lungs might end up in the bones, liver or brain.

- **Hijack normal tissue:** It doesn't just sit there. Cancer grows into organs and steals space, resources and nutrients like an invasive species destroying a delicate ecosystem.

Essentially, cancer doesn't kill you directly. Cruelly, it makes your organs unable to function properly until they give up.

Talking about cancer

The language around cancer matters. Words can influence how we view things; they can capture our attention or alter our emotional response or interpretation of the world around us.

Some languages assign grammatical gender to inanimate objects. French, Spanish, Italian and German (among others) have long maintained this grammatical quirk, where nouns are categorised as masculine, feminine or neuter. If an object is masculine in their language, they're more likely to use 'strong' or 'hard' adjectives. If it's feminine, they'll lean toward softer, more elegant descriptors.

Let's take death (*la muerte* in Spanish; *der tod* in German). In Spanish, death is feminine and so in Spanish literature she often appears as a veiled, mysterious woman. But in Germany, where death is masculine, he's more likely to show up as a grim reaper with a scythe, ready to collect his due like an old-school tax collector. Or consider a car (*el coche*, which is masculine, in Spanish; *la voiture*, feminine, in French). The Spanish masculine car evokes descriptions of power, speed and robustness, while the French feminine car is more likely to be described in terms of elegance, beauty and design.

So what does this have to do with cancer? Well, in much the same way, the types of words we use to talk about cancer can shape the way we interact or respond to it. The right language can help to prevent stereotypes or misinformation and even make someone's life easier if they're going through cancer.

The Big C

Cancer isn't the biggest killer of humans (that award goes to cardiovascular disease), but it provokes a far greater emotional response. When someone dies of a heart attack, we don't say they 'lost a battle with heart disease'. Similarly, someone who recovers from a stroke is rarely described as a 'stroke survivor', as would a cancer survivor, despite strokes leaving millions dead or disabled every year.

One fascinating study from 2019 showed that when cancer was viewed as an 'enemy' to be beaten, patients went along with more aggressive treatment as opposed to those who viewed cancer as a 'journey'. For some patients, the military metaphor helps to keep them motivated or determined, whereas for others, it places too much pressure on the patient to feel 'strong' or make them feel they didn't 'fight' hard enough in the face of cancer.

It's not uncommon also for people to be blamed for their cancer because of their supposed unhealthy lifestyle, sexual promiscuity or as a type of divine punishment or bad karma for past wrongdoings. By doing this, cancer becomes a taboo subject, something that should be hidden.

When I was a medical student shadowing senior doctors in clinics, I often noticed them using euphemisms for cancer and words like 'lump', 'abnormality' or 'growth' were frequently used. It felt dishonest and, while the intent might have been to avoid psychological distress and to soften the blow of an uncomfortable truth, it ultimately did not help. If anything, beating about the bush in this way simply allowed the patients' minds to run wild and assume the worst, needlessly causing further panic.

We should be having, not avoiding, conversations about cancer because the truth is many cancers, when caught early, are highly curable, with survival rates over 98 per cent for certain skin, breast, prostate, testicular and thyroid cancers. Let me repeat that. The word cancer does not mean a death sentence. We may never find the perfect language for cancer and the right message will vary depending on the patient, their own personal beliefs, the type of cancer and even depending on cultural context.

Shrouding the subject of cancer in mystery or shame will only provoke fear and deter people from dealing with any early symptoms, leading to late diagnoses and poorer survival outcomes. Our taboo of cancer can literally kill.

Cancer: An age-old problem

Cancer is not a new disease. It has been detected and managed (with questionable outcomes in some cases) throughout history, from blood-letting, herbal remedies and arsenic pastes to primitive surgery involving cauterisation and the removal of lumps.

Up until the twentieth century, however, other diseases, such as tuberculosis, diphtheria, smallpox and influenza, took more of the limelight as in the days before antibiotics or vaccines they could spread quickly and kill in massive numbers. Most people didn't live long enough to develop cancer and if they did they were probably unaware they had it as it was far less visible than, say, the pustules of bubonic plague, which wiped out a third of the population in Europe in the Middle Ages.

When people started to live longer, as happened in the early part of the twentieth century, cancer went from the eighth to the second most common cause of death just behind heart disease – and has remained there ever since. The truth about our new longevity is that the longer we stick around on this mortal coil, the more chance we have of developing some form of cancer. In fact, if we all were to live long enough, it is likely that 100 per cent of humans (or very close to it) would get cancer.

As it is, over the course of our lives around 40 per cent of us are likely to develop it in some form or another. Even now, many people will have cancer without even knowing it and will die of something else first. As an example, autopsy studies have shown that half of men over sixty and three-quarters of those over seventy have undiagnosed prostate cancer. You're far more likely to die *with* prostate cancer than *of* it.

The Big C

> ### The tell-tale signs of cancer
>
> There are a few tried and tested symptoms we can look out for when it comes to cancer. This is a very rough guide and by no means exhaustive. Indeed, many of the symptoms here are associated with non-cancerous conditions, but any symptoms should still be examined to be safe. Similarly, there are some cancer symptoms, such as unexplained weight loss or fatigue, that aren't included in this easy-to-remember acronym created by the American Cancer Society:
>
> **C** – Change in bowel or bladder symptoms
> **A** – A non-healing sore
> **U** – Unusual or unexpected bleeding or discharge
> **T** – Thickening or lump in a part of the body
> **I** – Indigestion or trouble swallowing
> **O** – Overt or obvious change in a mole or mark
> **N** – Nagging or persistent cough or change in voice.

A pyrrhic victory?

Throughout my time as a doctor and surgeon, I've been involved in operations to remove cancers from all manner of body parts: breasts, skin, livers, colons, small intestines, stomachs, oesophagi, gallbladders, pancreases, spleens, rectums, appendixes and more. What's struck me most is that cancer is unrelenting. Treating cancer is not easy and often comes at significant cost to the patient. Cancer does yield when struck with surgery or powerful chemotherapy agents, but it can also lie dormant, gathering and regrouping before returning months or years later.

It sounds farcical, but in a sense, cancer seems to be a sentient being. It is selfish as, unlike normal human cells, which follow and obey instructions, cancer cells do what they need to do to flourish and act in their own best interests. Cancer also seemingly 'evolves'. It evades detection from the immune system, hides from medication, develops resistance to treatment, turns other cells into allies and can even lay low for years, waiting for the opportune moment to return to action. Like a cockroach, it is hard to kill.

Analogies aside, the scientist in me knows they aren't malevolent creatures. They are cells driven by the purpose of cells, to survive. And they do it well. Cancer is the price we pay for the years of evolution and renewing our cells.

Fighting back

Cancer treatments are a taboo within a taboo. We barely talk about cancer, and when we do, we whisper about chemotherapy and radiotherapy like they're medieval torture methods best left unspoken. The perception is that chemo makes you sick, radiotherapy sounds like nuclear warfare, and both are designed to ruin your quality of life before they save it.

And that's exactly why we need to talk about them. Because the fear of treatment is sometimes bigger than the fear of the disease itself. And that can be deadly.

Let's demystify what's actually happening at the cellular level, what these treatments *really* do, and whether every cancer patient is doomed to a bald, vomit-filled existence.

1. Chemotherapy: a sometimes necessary poison

Chemotherapy is the mother of all cancer treatments, the one most people have heard of, and the one that inspires the most dread. The simplified premise is: poison the cancer before it kills you.

At its core, chemotherapy is cytotoxic therapy, which means it's designed to kill fast-dividing cells. Cancer cells divide uncontrollably, so chemo is like a biological sniper targeting anything that's growing too quickly. But here's the problem: your body has other fast-dividing cells that aren't cancer.

- Hair follicles (hence the hair loss, but not *always*)
- Gut lining (which is why nausea and diarrhoea often come with the package)
- Bone marrow cells (leading to fatigue and lowered immunity).

So yes, chemo is brutal, but it's also highly strategic. It doesn't *just* obliterate cells randomly; it specifically goes after rapidly dividing ones.

Myths about chemotherapy

Myth: *Chemo always makes you bald.*

Not necessarily. Some types of chemo are more aggressive on hair follicles than others. There are also cooling caps now that can reduce hair loss by constricting blood vessels in the scalp.

Myth: *Chemo = constant vomiting.*

This was true once upon a time. But modern anti-nausea medication is so good that many patients feel mild nausea at most.

Myth: *You should avoid all food additives and live off kale and good karma while on chemo.*

No. You need protein, calories and actual sustenance to help your body recover. Chemo patients often struggle to maintain weight, so the priority is eating what you can tolerate, not obsessing over a 'clean' diet.

2. Radiotherapy: shooting cancer with science beams

If chemo is chemical warfare, radiotherapy is sniper fire. It uses high-energy radiation to fry cancer cells, damaging their DNA so they can't keep dividing. The body then naturally clears out the wreckage.

But here's the cool part: radiotherapy can be ridiculously precise. Unlike chemo, which affects the whole body, radiotherapy can target specific areas, meaning fewer side effects for many patients.

How does it work?

External beam radiation: A big scary machine that looks like something out of *Star Wars* directs radiation at a tumour from outside the body.

Internal radiation (brachytherapy): Tiny radioactive implants are placed inside the body, close to the tumour, like little radioactive spies infiltrating enemy lines.

Myths about radiotherapy

Myth: *You become radioactive.*

If you had external beam radiotherapy, you are *not* radioactive. You can hug your kids and pet your dog immediately. But if you've had internal radiotherapy (like brachytherapy), you *might* have temporary restrictions on close physical contact.

Myth: *It burns your skin off.*

Not quite. Some people experience mild skin irritation, but it's usually localised and manageable, not third-degree sci-fi burns.

3. Targeted therapy: the sniper that doesn't miss

Targeted therapies attack cancer on a molecular level, focusing on specific proteins or mutations that fuel tumour growth. Unlike chemo, which goes after any fast-dividing cell, targeted therapies are designed to leave normal cells alone, meaning fewer side effects.

Example: HER2-positive breast cancer can be treated with Herceptin, a drug that blocks the HER2 protein and stops tumour growth without nuking every fast-dividing cell in sight.

4. Immunotherapy: teaching your own body to fight back

Your immune system already knows how to kill rogue cells, it just sucks at recognising cancer because tumours develop cloaking devices.

The Big C

Immunotherapy works by removing those disguises and letting your body's natural defence system go full John Wick on cancer cells.

Checkpoint inhibitors (like Keytruda) remove the 'brakes' from immune cells, allowing them to attack cancer more aggressively.

CAR-T therapy is like giving your immune system a PhD in cancer-killing. It genetically engineers your T-cells to recognise and destroy specific tumours.

Warnings: the stuff they don't tell you (but should)

Toilet rules: If you're on chemo, your fluids are toxic (at least briefly). Once chemotherapy is done killing cancer, it comes out in your bodily fluids. That means:

- Flush twice after using the toilet
- If you live with others, clean the seat and lid thoroughly
- If you menstruate, dispose of pads/tampons carefully (double-bag them)
- If you're sexually active, use protection. Some chemo drugs linger in bodily fluids and can be passed on to your partner.
- Avoid sick people like they have the plague (because they might). Chemo suppresses your immune system, so a normal cold for someone else could land you in the hospital.
- Wash your hands religiously
- Avoid large crowds during flu season
- Don't let people 'power through' their colds near you.

Yes, chemo and radiotherapy can be rough. But they are also incredibly effective, and they have evolved far beyond the horror stories we heard in decades past. The real danger isn't the treatment; it's avoiding the conversation. Fear and misinformation stop people from getting screened, from starting therapy, from knowing what to expect.

Cancer isn't Voldemort and it doesn't get stronger if we say its name. Nor do chemotherapy, radiotherapy or immunotherapy. The more we understand them, the less power fear has over us.

So, if you or someone you love is facing cancer, talk about it. Ask questions. Learn. Because knowledge, not silence, is the most powerful weapon we have.

Cancerphobia

We live in an age where seemingly everything causes cancer. Media headlines sound alarm bells around pesticides, food additives and modern products such as synthetic plastics.

Despite good evidence – which suggests that the bulk of cancers are a result of natural processes that can lead to DNA mutations, which then cause uncontrolled cell proliferation in addition to the role that various lifestyle factors play in reducing cancer risk (to a tune of 40 per cent reduction) – the myth remains entrenched that cancer is a result of modern vices and our modern environment.

This myth is in part propagated by media outlets and suggests that 'in antiquity' (science-speak for a long time ago) cancer was scarce in the ancient world and is, in fact, a disease of modern excesses.

Do we have carcinogenic environmental factors that cause cancer? Yes. But so did the ancients. Most of these quips about cancer being virtually non-existent in a bygone era is because people 'in antiquity' didn't live long enough to get it, and the high prevalence of cancer in the modern era is an unhappy by-product of our lengthier lifespans. It's also worth noting that cancer of the soft tissue (such as bowel cancer) does not show up in fossils.

It can be psychologically taxing to constantly have to worry about the dozens of things we interact with in our daily lives that *could* have a risk of cancer and which are largely out of our control. But we have decades of research that clearly show that a limited number of things which *are* mostly well within our control have the most important role in influencing our cancer risk; these are not smoking, keeping a healthy weight, limiting or avoiding alcohol, getting enough exercise and avoiding sunburn.

Chimney sweeps

In 1775, the eminent English surgeon Percivall Pott published a pivotal paper about chimney sweeps and scrotums. You must be wondering why this piece of research was so seminal (excuse the multilayered pun here)? It was, in fact, the first time an environmental agent had been identified as carcinogenic (having the potential to cause cancer).

Pott had observed an abnormally high incidence of scrotal cancer in chimney sweeps and suggested that the cause was exposure to soot, which accumulated on their skin as they crawled up narrow chimneys.

Not all chimney sweeps developed cancer but it transpired that the ones who worked more often were more likely to be exposed to carcinogens, thus increasing their cancer risk, a vital contribution to our understanding of cancer.

This may seem obvious to a modern reader: your skin cancer risk will be naturally higher if you sunbathe for ten hours a day on a sun-soaked Australian beach versus going for a thirty-minute outdoor walk during a soggy Canadian winter. Conversely, why is it that some people who smoke or who are exposed to carcinogens on a daily basis don't get cancer?

Your body has an in-built auto-repair function – to a degree. DNA damage (up to a certain point) can be repaired naturally by the body, although there will be a point or threshold at which carcinogens can cause irreversible harm. This threshold will vary from person to person and is influenced in part by genetics, health and diet (antioxidants in fruit and vegetables for example).

This Is Vital Information

The IARC and carcinogens

Thanks to child labour laws and central heating, we rarely send children up chimneys these days, thereby reducing exposure to the carcinogen of soot. However, there are numerous other substances that could cause cancer and require vigilance. The most widely acknowledged and referenced classification for carcinogens is from the International Agency for Research on Cancer, or IARC.

Group 1. There is enough evidence to conclude that these carcinogens cause cancer in humans. Substances or agents include tobacco, benzene (a liquid found in coal tar and petroleum), asbestos, UV light and alcohol. Occupations are also included in the list, and painters and cabinetmakers are included in group 1 owing to their exposure to solvents, wood dust and other carcinogenic substances. Once again, the amount of exposure to these substances is key – a large majority of the world consume alcohol but might not develop cancer.

Group 2A is a list of 'probable' carcinogens and the evidence here comes primarily from animal studies, with some limited human studies. Substances include acrylamide in burned food items, baked items, chemicals from some lines of work such as hairdressing, and, perhaps surprisingly, shift work (because of the disruption to circadian sleep patterns).

Group 2B contains the 'possibly carcinogenic' factors. This is based on limited animal and human studies and this is where things get interesting. This list contains things like coffee, fermented vegetables – both of which have powerful antioxidant potential and have positive influences on gut health and the microbiome, which, counterintuitively, we know can also *reduce* cancer risk. Sometimes it feels like you just can't win.

The three groups, in fact, list more than 450 substances or items as known, probable or possible carcinogens. Often, the mere inclusion of a substance in any of these categories – even on the 'possible' list – is enough to cause significant concern and confusion among the public. I mean we are encouraged to eat fermented food and pickled vegetables because they're good for our gut health but it's also a possible carcinogen?

The issue is that the IARC evaluation is based on hazard. Pickled vegetables can indeed cause cancer in some animals when they're exposed to phenomenally high concentrations. This is enough for the IARC to label such substances as carcinogenic. However, if you perform a risk analysis rather than a hazard analysis – evaluating the risk of getting cancer in real life, under realistic exposure levels – suddenly the substances appear to be far safer.

In 2015, the IARC created pandemonium when it labelled processed meats as a group 1 carcinogen. Based on 800 publications, the IARC estimated that if a person ate 50g of processed meat daily, in a lifetime this leads to an increased cancer risk of 18 per cent.

For an individual, then, the risk over a lifetime of eating processed meats is about 1 in 100. On an individual level that might be a small risk, but on an epidemiological level, with millions of people eating only processed meats, the population-level impact can be significant. The IARC estimated there were around 34,000 cases per year.

But is all this data actually helpful? It is physically impossible to avoid every known or suspected carcinogen? That doesn't mean we shouldn't try to avoid the worst offenders – I'd lose my medical licence if I advised you to throw caution to the wind and start smoking a pack of cigarettes a day – but equally we shouldn't avoid leaving the house for fear of crossing paths with a cabinetmaker.

Focus on what is in your control to ensure your 'risk' of cancer is reduced. Limit alcohol intake, wear sunscreen to protect against excessive UV radiation, avoid smoking, limit or avoid processed meats, increase activity levels, consume fruits and vegetables, which will help to support the repair mechanism of your DNA. And, of course, never, ever become a chimney sweep.

This Is Vital Information

> *Testicular cancer: the curable epidemic we're too embarrassed to beat*
>
> Humans will boldly TikTok their deepest insecurities, but ask them to check their balls for life-saving clues? Sounds sus. Testicular cancer is the most curable solid tumour when caught early (with a 95 per cent survival rate) but we'd rather risk metastasis than admit our scrotums might need a doctor's glance. One in 250 men will develop it, yet 35 per cent delay care because of shame.

The anatomy of embarrassment

Testicles are evolutionary marvels – sperm factories dangling in a climate-controlled sac (scrotum) governed by the dartos muscle. This fleshy thermostat tightens in cold, relaxes in warmth. Hence the shower examination hack: warm water loosens the dartos, making lumps feel like 'a pea in a water balloon' versus 'a pea in a sock'. Yet even this fails to motivate men to grope their own gonads monthly. Thanks to a blend of toxic masculinity (real men don't get sick), sexual insecurities (fears equating losing a testicle with losing one's manhood) and society's prudishness around everything in that general area, too many men simply don't know how to check their balls.

So men die of treatable tumours because they'd rather meme about 'big dick energy' than confront a small dick anomaly.

Symptoms: your balls' cry for help

Your testicles don't subtweet or post Instagram reels. They give you biological clues that you should get checked out by a doctor.

- **'Heavy scrotum':** Feels like lugging a walnut in a sock filled with lead.

- **'Lump'**: Not the 'gainz' you want. Could be smooth (spermatocele) or gritty (tumour).
- **'Ache'**: Dull throbs in the groin or lower back (lymph node metastasis waving 'Hi!').

How to fondle your balls:

- **Monthly ball audit:** Give your balls a feel at least once a month.
- **Shower time:** Warm water relaxes the dartos. Think 'avocado inspection' – gentle, systematic.
- **Roll, don't squeeze:** Thumb on top, fingers beneath. Glide over the testicle's surface. The epididymis (the back side) should feel like a tender noodle – normal.
- **If you find a lump:** Don't wait it out – go see a doctor.
- **Compare and despair:** If one testicle is larger than the other, don't worry. Asymmetry is natural. Rocks ≠ raisins.

Billions of years of cosmic evolution led to this moment: *you*, avoiding a mirror to check for lumps because society said balls = pride. Now go forth and check your bollocks in the name of medicine.

The future of cancer

In the past, cancer was deemed a death sentence, whereas now for many people it is a chronic disease and survivable; especially if your bank balance is considerably hefty.

Cancer screening and better treatments are increasingly available across the globe, but access remains uneven, reflecting deep inequalities. As the socio-economic divide between those with money and those without continues to grow, so does the disparity of cancer mortality rates.

In the US, the death rate for cancer has plummeted by 27 per cent, from 215 deaths per 100,000 people in 1991 to 156 per 100,000 in 2016. Better detection and treatment is making cancer more survivable. Indeed, in 2018 the *Lancet* published one of the largest studies of cancer survival trends (in seventy-one countries and 67 per cent of the world's population from 2000 to 2014) and found cancer survival was increasing in many countries.

The other part of the story is to do with prevention. Public health policies – giving advice on stopping smoking and campaigns to curb cancer-causing activities – have also contributed to a decline in cancer death rates.

But similar success was not seen everywhere in the world and where you live influences your chances of overcoming cancer. For childhood brain cancers, the five-year survival rate in Scandinavian countries is about 80 per cent. Shockingly, though, this number drops to under 40 per cent in countries like Brazil and Mexico. These disparities are even more marked within different socio-economic backgrounds within the same country. One study in 2017 showed that Americans with a high income bracket are up to three times less likely to die of lung or bowel cancer than their poorer counterparts. Worryingly, these gaps in health outcomes continue to widen.

Socio-economic status impacts access to healthcare – due to poor healthcare facilities, lack of awareness or myriad other factors – which in turn affects cancer survival chances. Without access to adequate cancer screening, the odds are the disease won't be diagnosed until a much later stage, when the chances of survival are much lower.

Adopting a lifestyle that can help prevent the onset of cancer is also key, but inequalities here also exist. It's far easier to eat well and make it to the gym regularly when you're not worrying about keeping a roof over your head. A 2016 study analysing US income data and mortality rates between 1999 and 2014 found a significant gap in life expectancy between the richest and the poorest. Men in the top 1 per cent of earners lived fifteen years longer than men in the bottom 1 per cent. For women the gap was ten years. Money is not the only driving factor as people on low incomes who lived in affluent, better-educated areas were more likely to adopt healthier lifestyles and consequently lived longer than people with the same income living in poorer, less well-educated neighbourhoods. While these figures are not specific to cancer, they show the inequalities embedded in healthcare systems, of which cancer treatment forms a key part.

Why we can't cure cancer

The problem with this lofty aim is that it assumes we can create a magic bullet of sorts that can eliminate the burden of cancer in its entirety. In truth, we need to focus more on prevention as the cure, or change our perception of the word cure.

Right now, we are a million miles from a 'cure'. This moonshot idea is based on a premise that cancer is one disease, when in fact the word cancer is merely a term for a plethora of diseases, each having its own unique genetic fingerprint, cause and pathology.

The reduction in cancer mortality we've seen over the last few decades is in large part down to public health measures and cancer prevention interventions such as colonoscopies and mammograph screenings, as well as the roll-out of vaccinations (notably hepatitis B, hepatitis C and HPV).

Some of these preventative strategies can 'cure' cancer by eliminating some of the worst ones from materialising in the first place. Hepatocellular carcinoma, or liver cancer, is the third most common cause of cancer mortality in the world and is caused in the main by the hepatitis C viruses. If you are infected with hep C you have seventeen-times greater risk of getting liver cancer. If only every government would pay attention.

Cancer prevention: a call to arms

If cancer were a foreign enemy, governments would have declared war on it centuries ago. It would have been the subject of endless policy briefings, emergency summits and trillion-dollar defence budgets. There would be cancer response task forces, cancer intelligence agencies, and world leaders gravely delivering speeches about how we will not rest until we defeat this menace.

And yet, here we are, with one in two people expected to get cancer in their lifetime, and somehow, the global response remains half-hearted, disorganised, and weirdly reluctant to acknowledge the scale of the problem. If a contagious disease wiped out as many people as cancer does, the world would be in a full-blown panic. But cancer isn't contagious. It's just biological betrayal at its finest, so instead of a swift and aggressive response, we drag our feet, underfund research, and pretend kale is a sufficient defence strategy.

Where are we failing?

1. Prevention is an afterthought, not a priority

Governments love funding treatments, but they neglect prevention. This is the equivalent of putting out multiple fires without ever questioning the guy with matches standing nearby.

We know that lifestyle factors like smoking, diet, alcohol and air pollution contribute massively to cancer risk, yet for the most part, governments hesitate to regulate industries that profit from human self-destruction. The tobacco industry still thrives, junk food is marketed like it's a human right and carcinogens lurk in cosmetics, plastics and household chemicals without proper scrutiny.

Prevention campaigns exist, sure, but they are woefully underfunded compared with the billions spent on treating late-stage disease or the money spent by lobbyists to protect these carcinogenic products.

2. Early detection is an afterthought too

If we caught cancer earlier, survival rates would skyrocket. But cancer screening programmes are patchy, underutilised, and often inaccessible to the people who need them most.

The Big C

Mammograms, colonoscopies, cervical screenings and PSA tests save lives. And yet governments are weirdly bad at getting people to actually have them. In 2024, over a third of women invited by the NHS to breast screening appointments did not attend. In some countries, getting a routine scan is easier said than done. Delayed appointments, expensive procedures and bureaucratic hurdles make screening a luxury rather than a necessity.

Many low-income populations simply don't get screened, meaning cancer is caught late, survival is far lower and treatment costs skyrocket. People on low income often lack the health insurance needed to access screening, have less awareness about screenings or a mistrust of healthcare systems, or there are simply fewer facilities where they live.

3. Big pharma needs more transparency

New cancer drugs cost obscene amounts of money, ensuring that access is a privilege, not a right. In countries without subsidised healthcare, some patients can't afford life-saving treatments while pharma CEOs luxuriate in record-breaking bonuses.

We need radical drug pricing reform. In a just world, surviving cancer shouldn't come with a side effect of financial ruin.

4. Healthcare systems are failing patients

Cancer care is only as good as the system delivering it. And in many places, that system is a dysfunctional, underfunded, bureaucratic mess.

Countries with universal healthcare at least ensure that everyone gets access, but delays, shortages and inefficiencies still cost lives. In nations without universal healthcare (*cough*, the US, *cough*), your survival literally depends on your bank account. Long wait times and overburdened hospitals mean that many patients aren't getting the best possible care simply because there aren't enough resources.

This Is Vital Information

So what needs to happen?

If we want to 'beat' cancer, governments need to treat prevention like a national security issue. The way forward is clear but we need our politicians to do something about it.

- **Regulate known carcinogens:** Tobacco, junk food, air pollution and other carcinogens should be regulated not just with weak public service announcements, but with actual laws.

- **Put money into public health campaigns** that make early detection as automatic as brushing your teeth.

- **Make screenings easy to access and free**, and aggressively promote them. No one should have to jump through hoops to get a mammogram, colonoscopy or Pap smear. Bring screenings to workplaces, homes and underserved communities.

- **Make Big Pharma accountable:** We need transparent pricing, fair drug costs and investment in actual cures, not just expensive treatments. Government-funded cancer research should favour non-profitable solutions, because leaving cancer cures to corporations is a clear conflict of interest.

- **Ensure hospitals have adequate funds**, employ more oncologists and enable faster access to life-saving treatments. Ensure cancer care is accessible to all, not just the wealthy or well-insured.

In the end, cancer doesn't care if you ignore it. It doesn't care if it makes you uncomfortable. It doesn't care if you're busy, uninsured or too afraid to book that screening.

Governments, institutions and corporations need to be held accountable, but as individuals, we also need to stop waiting for the cavalry to arrive. Get screened. Encourage others to get screened. Call out bad policies. Demand action.

The Big C

The great MRI debate

The golden rule of cancer is that if you catch it early, you improve your chances of treating it before it becomes catastrophic. That applies also to cardiovascular health, and basically all of medicine: early detection = better survival.

In an era where people track their REM sleep with military precision, count their steps like they're hoarding currency in a dystopian sci-fi novel, and wear rings, watches and glucose monitors to study every biological squeak their body makes, why not (if you have the means) go for a full-body MRI (magnetic resonance imaging) scan. All you need to do is lie in a giant magnetic tube for just an hour or ninety minutes while it captures pictures of nearly all the major organs, tissues and structures across your whole body and spend several thousand dollars!

Celebrities like Kim Kardashian, Jeff Bezos and a parade of billionaires have publicly praised them. The idea of catching something early before it 'becomes a problem' is seductive. Technology makes us feel empowered. After all, if we can monitor everything else, why not scan the whole damn body while we're at it?

So, at face value, the logic behind a full-body MRI is compelling. Let's look at the pros and cons.

Pro: It gives you peace of mind. If the scan finds absolutely nothing, congratulations. You have the biological equivalent of a verified blue tick on Twitter.

Pro: It *might* catch something that would otherwise have been missed. We're talking early-stage cancer, an aneurysm or a weird structural anomaly. Finding one before it's a crisis could literally save your life.

Pro: It's not just about disease. Some people just want to know everything about their own body. What if you have a funky kidney shape? What if you have a tiny benign brain cyst that means nothing but sounds cool to tell people about?

This Is Vital Information

MRI is like getting a Google Earth scan of your insides. And in an age where we are obsessed with tracking every aspect of our health, this seems like the next logical step.

But there are disadvantages to full-body MRIs – it's not like getting a routine check-up. They are sensitive, prone to false positives and, in many cases, lead to more harm than good.

Con: Incidentalomas (aka the rabbit hole of doom). Most people have weird stuff inside them, whether that's a small nodule in the lung, a harmless cyst or an asymmetrical structure that means nothing. A full-body MRI finds these things, and suddenly you're in a cycle of unnecessary follow-ups, biopsies and stress. If you scan 100 asymptomatic people, a huge number will have 'findings' that are completely meaningless. But now, you're googling obscure diseases and assuming you have two weeks to live.

Con: False positives and unnecessary procedures. A small, benign cyst might be flagged as suspicious, leading to a biopsy. The biopsy might lead to complications, infections or unnecessary surgeries. One 'abnormality' turns into six months of extra testing, hospital visits and stress for something that was never going to harm you.

Con: The accuracy problem (not as good as you think). Screening tests need high sensitivity (so they catch real diseases) and high specificity (so they don't catch fake problems). Full-body MRIs are not tuned for specific cancers, so they are neither sensitive enough nor specific enough to be reliable for population-wide screening.

For comparison, mammograms work because breast cancer is common, the tech is fine-tuned and we know what to look for. Full-body MRIs? They are looking for anything and everything. Which means lots of noise, lots of confusion and lots of unnecessary anxiety.

The verdict

If you have a strong family history of cancer, an undiagnosed mystery illness, or can actually afford to throw down thousands for peace of mind, then sure, get a full-body MRI. It might find something. But for the average, healthy person? It's expensive, anxiety-inducing and statistically more likely to lead to unnecessary stress than actual life-saving discoveries.

So what should you do instead?

- Stick to screenings with proven benefits (mammograms, colonoscopies, Pap smears).
- Prioritise lifestyle factors such as sleep, diet, exercise, avoiding carcinogens.
- If you're genuinely worried, talk to an actual doctor – and not a billionaire on Instagram.

Yes, the distrust in the healthcare system is real. Yes, we all want control over our own health. But more data isn't always better. And sometimes, knowing too much can be just as dangerous.

Chapter 10

DEATH 2.0

I MUST WARN YOU THAT the following pages contain details you might find distressing. It is about death, after all.

You never know when such a day will hit. I had some forewarning of this event, but the impact was nonetheless still unexpectedly severe.

In 2007, I was in the midst of revising for my fifth-year medical school exams as well as doing clinical rotations. My grandmother, who I had been very close to since I was a child, had just been admitted to hospital with a blood clot in her lungs. The treatment for this involves using a blood thinner to stop the clot from progressing. Unfortunately, the doctors had over-anticoagulated her, causing her to bleed internally.

All this was happening in a hospital thousands of miles away in India. Stuck in London, I was receiving daily updates from my dad, who had flown out to be by her side. I was ready to throw everything away. *Screw the exams*, I thought to myself. *I want to be with Ajji.* But my parents insisted she would not have wanted me to discard a career I had worked so hard for. By completing medical school, they reminded me, I would continue to make her proud.

Shortly afterwards, coming home after finishing a day of clinical rotations, my mum was waiting for me.

'Ajji's gone,' she said simply.

This Is Vital Information

It was the first time in my life that I felt such overwhelming despair and anguish. You know the Hollywood movie trope, where the protagonist falls to their knees after hearing of a tragedy? Turns out that's a stereotype for a reason. I found myself in a similar stance, with tears flooding down my face and flitting between crying and screams of anger, frustration and self-pity.

Since that day, I've delivered similar bad news to countless patients and relatives, from cancer diagnoses to death, failed treatments and unexpected events that could turn someone's life upside down. Yet, the little that medical school had taught me about breaking bad news was, to put it politely, awful.

The very first time I had to tell a family that their father had passed away, I tried to use the template I had been given as a student. It was blunt, heavy-handed and clumsy, three things you don't want when having an end-of-life or bad-news conversation. And like all the most embarrassing moments in life, I remember it like it was yesterday.

The template I was given wasn't much more than 'Hello, I'm Dr [Insert Name]. I'm so sorry for your loss' and 'Would you like me to get you some water?' But they don't teach you what to do when the family is staring at you with a mixture of sadness, anger, pain, shock – and the rest.

The gold standard of breaking bad news is now the SPIKES protocol, which was first published in 2000 as a way to give bad news to cancer patients and since then has been adopted more widely. It's a structured, compassionate, step-by-step guide to delivering awful, life-altering information with dignity. And, in theory, it sounds great.

- **S – Setting:** Private room, calm environment, tissues on standby
- **P – Perception:** 'What do you already understand about what's happening?'
- **I – Invitation:** 'Would you like me to explain more?'
- **K – Knowledge:** 'I'm afraid I have some difficult news . . .'

Death 2.0

- **E – Empathy:** 'I can only imagine how painful this must be.'
- **S – Summary and strategy:** Summarise the information and offer plan for next steps. 'Is there anyone I can call for you?'

Sounds nice, doesn't it? Clean. Professional. Human, but not *too* human.

So, with the confidence of a medical school graduate who had never actually done this before, I walked into the room, sat down and prepared to deliver my pre-rehearsed, robotic masterpiece of compassionate communication.

I started strong. 'I'm so sorry . . . your father has passed away.'

Silence. A long, gut-wrenching, soul-crushing silence where time stood still and the air in the room became suffocating. And then my mouth – uncontrollably, catastrophically – decided that silence was the enemy.

I filled it with words. Too many words.

'Uh . . . he . . . he was very peaceful. He wasn't in pain. Well, I mean, we obviously can't ask him, but from what we observed . . . medically speaking . . . he looked comfortable. Well, as comfortable as one can be, you know, in a situation where they're . . . no longer . . . um . . . alive.'

I wanted to die. Not metaphorically. I genuinely wanted to cease existing in that moment. The family just stared at me in horror. Or confusion. Possibly both. At one point I think I offered them tea three times in one sentence.

'Would you like some tea? Water? Or, well, tea? We also have tea?'

I was so deep in panic mode that when one of the family members finally said: 'Are you sure?' I almost responded with: 'Yes. I checked.'

Luckily, my last remaining brain cell activated just in time, preventing me from actually saying that out loud. Instead, I nodded sombrely, shut up for once and let them grieve.

Lesson learned: death is not a moment. It's a vacuum. And in that vacuum, words don't work the way you think they will. No amount of preparation in a lecture hall can teach you how to sit with someone's grief in real-time.

I left that room feeling like I had failed the family, the patient, and every single communication skills seminar I had ever sat through.

But here's the thing about being a doctor: you only get better by first being bad. Since then, I've had hundreds of these conversations. I know when to speak and when to be silent. I know how to be fully present, rather than grasping at words to fill the void. I know now that breaking bad news is not about delivering a script. It's about absorbing someone else's world crashing down and standing with them in that moment.

And most importantly? I've learned how to offer tea just once.

TALKING ABOUT DEATH

So, how *should* you tell someone that their loved one has died? Surely this monumental moment deserves more than an algorithmic response?

In ten years working as a doctor, I've come to the conclusion that too often the medical field likes to cloak and obscure truths in medical language because we think it will be easier for the patient to hear. Everything is delivered through a professional filter to become less direct, more impersonal. In my experience, however, I think the most compassionate way to break bad news is to let the facts speak for themselves and to give space and time for that individual to process what it means to them.

As humans, we don't like to talk about death. It's the ultimate taboo, because to discuss it is to confront our own mortality. The catch is that by not talking about death we can become fearful of it, and frankly life's just too short for that.

Most of us don't think about death every day – which is perfectly logical. Death isn't nice and it comes with feelings of misery and sorrow. So, what fathomable reason would there be for making it a regular fixture in our thoughts?

Death 2.0

As a result, instead of dwelling on death, we distract ourselves with all manner of things, 'burying existential anxieties under a mound of French fries', as the social psychologist Sheldon Solomon puts it, comforting ourselves with delicious fast food rather than distinctly unappetising notions of death.

There are, however, some surprising benefits to spending more time thinking about death. Some psychological studies have found that mortality salience (basically dwelling on the subject) can raise an individual's sense of self-worth and encourage them to be less materialistic. Allegedly, it can also make them funnier (naturally, I think about it *all the time*).

With findings like this, it's no surprise that death cafés (yes, it's a thing) have become increasingly popular spaces for people to freely discuss the inevitable. These are social spaces where people can discuss their mortality over a cup of coffee, mirroring traditional Eastern religions that have death-centric thoughts and considerations rooted in their philosophies. Indeed, an ancient practice in Buddhism is to meditate on a corpse as it goes through the various stages of decomposition. The purpose is to contemplate the inevitability of death and to deepen appreciation and gratitude for human life.

Now that we're thinking about death, we should probably think about what it actually entails. And I suggest you banish all thoughts of those French fries, because it's time to talk about decomposition.

Let's break it down

Most of us have very little idea about what happens to the body after death. I'll warn you that what follows is morbid, to say the least, but my hope is that by understanding exactly what lies in store for us all, you might find that there is some beauty in these darkest moments.

I vividly remember when I was called to the hospital mortuary to see a recently deceased patient. Hospital policy required a medical doctor to review the bodies and check them for pacemakers or internal cardiac devices, which could explode during cremation.

I wandered into the bowels of the hospital and along the dark corridors I would get to know well over the subsequent years.

The mortuary technician checked me in and opened what was essentially a large steel drawer. Inside the figure of a body wrapped in a white cloth was clearly visible. Peeling back the cloth, I saw the purplish-grey skin of the patient – a sign that the early stages of decomposition had begun. The skin was cold to the touch and felt slightly wet.

Paradoxically, while the light may have been extinguished from this patient's eyes, inside there was still a lot going on. A corpse is teeming with life, a complex ecosystem that bursts into activity after death, driving the natural march of decomposition.

First, within a few minutes of death, autolysis begins. Once the heart stops beating, the cells are deprived of oxygen and enzymes inside the cells begin to break down the cell membranes to trigger a prison break. Red blood cells and blood vessels then begin to rupture and coalesce to discolour the skin.

The moment you die, your body also does something unexpected – it relaxes completely. It's called primary flaccidity and, for a brief window, your muscles are as limp as a badly made soufflé. It's a deceiving calm before the storm, because within two to six hours, the real fun begins.

The stiffening

The first time I encountered rigor mortis (the Latin term meaning 'stiffness of death') I was deeply unsettled. Death had always felt like a concept, a transition, an absence. But this? This was physical.

And yet, the moment wasn't entirely clinical. There's something profoundly humbling about seeing the body do its thing one last time; there's something unshakably human about it. Death is universal, but the body still follows its own rules, no matter who you are.

Death 2.0

Rigor mortis is the body's final act of defiance, a biochemical 'not today, Satan' moment where, for a few short hours, it refuses to go quietly into the night. During life, protein filaments in muscle cells facilitate contraction and relaxation of the muscles, but in death, there is no gas left in the tank for these proteins to do their work. If you've ever seen it in person, you'll know that death isn't instant stillness.

- **Two to six hours after death:** Rigor mortis starts setting in. Small muscles (the jaw, fingers, eyelids) begin to stiffen before it moves to the larger muscles. If someone dies mid-frown, their resting face is going to be very disappointed for a while.

- **Twelve hours after death:** Peak stiffness. The whole body has gone full statue mode. The limbs resist movement, joints become locked and everything feels unnervingly firm.

- **Twenty-four to forty-eight hours after death:** Rigor mortis slowly fades as enzymes and bacteria get to work. The body relaxes once more, this time permanently (well, until the decomposition party starts, but let's not get ahead of ourselves).

Imagine trying to bend a mannequin's arm that really doesn't want to be bent. That's rigor mortis. It's not unbreakable so if you really force it, you can move the limbs, but they'll resist with an unnerving amount of tension.

For forensic professionals, this stiffness helps them estimate time of death – though the process is affected by factors like temperature, muscle mass and cause of death. (Cold slows rigor down, heat speeds it up, and extreme muscle exertion before death can cause it to appear almost immediately.)

Some of you might have heard of something else that happens during rigor mortis – the final salute. It's called a priapism, or more poetically, 'angel lust'. For men who die in certain conditions (brain trauma, some poisons, hanging) the pelvic blood vessels collapse in a way that traps blood in the penis, resulting in a very final stiffy. It's awkward, it's absurd, and I'm sure somewhere out there, a forensic pathologist has had to explain it to a very confused family member.

The death microbiome

The cadaveric ecosystem at the point of death consists of a complex community of microscopic tenants that are already renting space in the human body. This is often referred to as the microbiome – a collection of bacteria, viruses and various microorganisms that live in or on the human body. The busiest neighbourhood, or most densely populated area, is in the gut – which is home to trillions of microbes.

The science and what we know about the microbiome is rapidly growing but we are still in the early stages, particularly when it comes to understanding what happens after death. In fact, the first study about the post-mortem microbiome wasn't published until 2014 so it's a relatively new and emerging field of research.

What we do know is that during life the microbiome is kept in check by the immune system. On death, the gut microbes, mostly in the form of bacteria, can spread freely and digest the prison that contains them – the intestines. These microscopic agents, which once used fibre as a fuel source, feed on chemicals leeching out of damaged cells. These microbes head off to nearby organs and tissues, like the liver and kidneys, and eventually the whole body.

Samples taken from corpses after death suggest that there may be some form of microbial clock that dictates the manner and speed in which bacteria systematically spread from organ to organ. This carefully choreographed takeover might provide a way for forensic scientists to estimate the time since death.

Bacterial-induced digestion (autodigestion) is followed by putrefaction. Twenty-four to seventy-two hours after death, early putrefaction begins as bacteria migrates from the gut to other organs.

Death 2.0

Between three and seven days, gases accumulate and over the next one to three weeks, soft tissue continues to break down into gases, liquids and component parts. As the bacteria feasts on the human carcass, gases such as methane and hydrogen sulphide are produced, which give a bloated appearance to the abdomen.

The increasing pressure created by these gases causes the skin to blister, loosen and outer layers may slip off. The gases attempt to break free from every available orifice, causing body cavities to rupture.

After around one to three weeks, as the cadaver 'opens' up, insects – such as blow flies, flesh flies and maggots – move in, accelerating the decay. They attract larger insects such as ants, wasps and spiders, which feed on the larvae and eggs of the flies. Progressively larger scavengers may join the party to partake in the feast of the body.

Three to six weeks after death, insect and microbial activity slows as a result of soft tissue loss, and the remaining cadaver decomposes, its various minerals and nutrients leeching into the soil and the circle of life continues. Death is just the beginning.

The five stages of bad science

When my grandmother died in the midst of my medical school exams, I didn't talk about it much with my parents or close friends. I suppressed the grief to take my exams and never tracked back to deal with it, even weeks and months later.

Grief is intertwined with the taboo of death and people don't like to talk about it beyond offering condolences or a tray of lasagne that will inevitably make its way into the bin a week later. Despite being something that will come to all of us, grief remains one of society's greatest taboos. We are allowed to grieve – but only briefly, quietly, and in ways that don't make anyone else uncomfortable. There's an unspoken deadline on mourning, and God help you if you exceed it. 'Aren't you over that yet?' 'Still sad?' 'Maybe you should get out more.'

This Is Vital Information

You are probably familiar with the 'five stages of grief': denial (this can't be happening); anger (why is this happening and who can I blame?); bargaining (maybe if I do this I can change the outcome); depression (there is no point in going on); and acceptance (it's happening and I will have to face it). These have been widely accepted as the stages people go through when grieving a loss.

Unfortunately, its widespread use is based on a pretty shaky premise. In the 1960s, the American psychiatrist Elisabeth Kübler-Ross conducted a series of interviews with terminally ill patients and created these five stages to describe the process they went through as they came to terms with their deaths. They were then applied to grieving friends and family, who seemed to go through a similar process. The problem was there was a lack of systematic analysis of Kübler-Ross's five stages, and little evidence to support the shift from basing it on the emotional experience of the dying to those mourning a loss.

It wasn't until the early 2000s that research from Yale University further explored the five stages of grief as part of the Yale Bereavement Study. Across a three-year period, they conducted 233 interviews with people who had lost a loved one. The study found that the emotional responses were complex and couldn't be broken down into five neatly defined stages. The incidence of denial was low and acceptance was the most prevalent emotion. The second strongest emotion was yearning or 'bargaining'. And their emotions didn't fit neatly into the five stages; they might skip or repeat stages or experience more than once; it wasn't a linear process.

Ultimately, there is no right or wrong way to grieve. No two people are alike, so how can we possibly expect them to react to death in the same way? People stricken by grief shouldn't be expected to feel a certain way or experience an arbitrary collection of emotions in a prescribed sequence. Grief changes over time, and everyone experiences it in their own individual way; at least that's what I've come to learn from my own losses and witnessing countless other grieving people in my work.

Death 2.0

Grief really does run deep – it's a biological, psychological and existential reconfiguration, a rewiring of everything you thought was stable. Your brain has to literally adapt to the absence of someone who once shaped your reality.

Neuroscience of grief: why it feels like you're losing your mind

When we bond with someone, our neurons weave them into the fabric of our mental universe. The prefrontal cortex, the part of the brain that governs reasoning, learns that 'this person exists' and expects to see them. The amygdala, our emotional processing centre, associates them with safety, comfort, love.

Then one day they're gone and your brain – still expecting their presence but not finding it – short-circuits. This is why grief feels like forgetting where you put your soul. Your brain is rewiring itself in real time, painstakingly unlearning a connection that once felt permanent.

So what should we do about it? What I've learned is that grief doesn't like silence. If you refuse to talk about it, it will find other ways to make itself heard, whether that's through your body, your dreams, your inability to focus, or your sudden irritability at small things (why did I just get emotionally overwhelmed by a packet of biscuits?).

You are not supposed to 'power through' grief, and shoving it into a mental cupboard with all your other unresolved traumas will not make it disappear. You need to talk about it. That doesn't mean giving an Oscar-worthy monologue about your sorrow to every passing stranger. But turn to your friends, family, a therapist, or even a support group. Let someone in.

Therapies like CBT (cognitive behavioural therapy) and ACT (acceptance and commitment therapy) have been shown to help process grief in a way that integrates it rather than suppresses it. Grief doesn't vanish, but it becomes something you can live with rather than something that dictates your every waking moment.

This Is Vital Information

Support groups also work. There is something profoundly comforting about sitting with others who just get it, without having to explain why you suddenly cried at a song that had no right to ambush you like that.

And if your usual instinct is to isolate? Try the opposite. There is no prize for suffering in silence. Reach out. Even if it's just to say 'Today was hard.' That's enough.

Talking about grief is the first step. The next? Talking about death itself. We plan for births, weddings, careers, retirement. But we treat death as something that should be ignored until it rudely interrupts us.

If grief teaches us anything, it's that we don't have as much time as we think we do. So maybe, instead of avoiding the subject entirely, we should learn to talk about it before it's too late. And if that thought makes you deeply uncomfortable, that's exactly why we need to start.

We're all in this together

When we look at nature and wildlife, death is ever-present. Animals are eaten alive; diseases ravage plant species; pathogens and microbes bring many things to their natural end. Death isn't an end point, it's a continuous, ongoing process that is simply an unavoidable part of living on Earth.

Despite this, few people have witnessed death first-hand – not even of an animal in the wild let alone another human being. When hospital patients are nearing the end of their life, they are sequestered into isolated side rooms away from the open wards, kept company only by the drones or trill of observation monitors or life-support machines providing the last vestiges of vital signs before they too go quiet. Death is concealed and sanitised.

The act of dying is often heavily medicalised, a condition that must be combatted rather than accepted as a natural life process. Those at the end of their lives who simply want to remain comfortable might, as a result of a family member, be kept alive unnaturally with the use of machines in the intensive care unit, or undergo complex surgery even though they are ninety-five years old with multiple conditions for which surgery may have no meaningful impact.

One of the consequences of the medicalisation of death is the belief that death is a personal responsibility – yours to deal with alone. If you die from a disease, it's your fault because of your unhealthy lifestyle, or it's a failure of your doctors to cure your affliction.

But why is this the case? If death is the great leveller, the one common thing that is experienced by every single person who has been or ever will be born, then why don't we view it as something to share, experience and even celebrate *together*?

I'm not suggesting you should obsess over death, rather the opposite. We know that countless survivors of near-death experiences have an overwhelming sense of elation. Perhaps the potent reminder of their proximity to death forces them to reappraise the price of every moment and how important it is to live with intent and purpose. Being reminded that life is limited increases its value.

You might have heard the Latin phrase 'carpe diem', or seize the day; grab life by its genitals, so to speak. But this abbreviated form of the sentence doesn't do its creator, the Roman poet Horace, justice. 'Carpe diem quam minimum credula postero' – 'Seize the day, never trust the next.'

Decisions, decisions

Every year in the UK, more than half a million people die. In most cases, it's from a disease or condition that gives some forewarning that death is on the way. My question to you is this: if you knew you didn't have long left, what would you do? Where would you want to meet your end? In a hospital or nursing home? A hospice? Who would you like to be with you? Doctors and healthcare staff or friends and family? Would you want major surgery? A ventilator to keep you breathing artificially for an undefined period of time, even if you're incredibly unlikely to regain consciousness?

This Is Vital Information

What is the limit, or the 'ceiling of care', that you would want treatment-wise? And do you have any thoughts either way on organ donation?

Too often people and families only consider what they want for the end of their life at the very last minute. At this point, however, many are unable to do that or are so incapacitated that they can no longer verbalise their wishes. As a result, their ending might not be exactly as they had wished.

But the good news about death, if I'm permitted to say such a thing, is that it is not always as bad as people think. It follows a somewhat predictable path in most cases. Illness and age reduce your energy levels to the point where more sleep is required, like an old battery running out of energy more quickly and requiring charging more frequently. The charging becomes progressively longer to the point where there may be occasional dips into unconsciousness until a point is reached where unconsciousness becomes the baseline.

Automatic breathing continues thanks to the functioning parts of the brain that control it, even if it does become shallow and noisy. Finally, there's an exhalation that isn't followed by an inhalation and that's that. It isn't always chaotic at the finish line, with excruciating pain or loss of control. This gentle death is what most people will experience.

So in light of this – do you know what your dying wishes are, and do your loved ones know what they are? It can, of course, be frightening to think about death and any suffering that might come with it. This is exactly why you need to prepare for death meticulously to ensure you have your goalposts clearly marked so things can go as close to plan as possible. This will also reduce the burden of difficult decision-making for your loved ones, who will also be going through an emotional time.

If someone is diagnosed with a chronic life-shortening disease or cancer, the timeframe between diagnosis and the finish line could be weeks, months or even years, giving at least some time to conclude unfinished business, plan for their own and families' future (property, wills, advanced directives and so on) and have all the conversations they need.

Death 2.0

But a sudden unexpected death robs a person and their family of that crucial planning time. Throughout my career I've dealt with situations where there is no plan in place from the patient's side about the type of care they want or crucially *not* want. Not every person wants to fight tooth and nail against the ravages of death and disease, especially if it involves invasive procedures that could leave them bed-bound for life or relying on artificial life-support systems for weeks or months. Many would prefer a comfortable, pain-free end, and not a long drawn-out battle against the inevitable.

Either way, if this isn't planned in advance, it is often difficult to establish how far the patient would want us to go with their care and we are often left making educated decisions based on medical necessity or a next of kin's assumption about what their relative would have wanted. Often, a family will want to do anything and everything to prevent death, which unbeknown to them might be against the true wishes of the patient in question.

The problem is the end isn't just an off switch. Sometimes the lead-up can be prolonged so it's important that any care or treatment aligns with the patient's wishes as much as possible.

Questions to think about might be: do you want to be admitted to the intensive care unit and have the full gamut of treatment including a ventilator? Would you want invasive feeding tubes in your nose, neck or stomach to nourish you with calorific and nutrient-dense liquid? How about comfort measures – would you prefer to be at home or in a hospice? Dying on your own terms, I've noticed, gives patients an extra layer of comfort and control when the process feels anything but controlled. You may even wish to appoint a proxy to make decisions in your stead. Making these decisions early prevents rushed, against-your-best-interest decisions when things take a sudden, unexpected turn for the worst.

To this day, I don't find having conversations about death easy, but I certainly feel more comfortable than I did as a freshly minted doctor many years ago. These end-of-life conversations can be awkward and unsettling if you're not used to them. Of course, this is a minor inconvenience when compared to the emotions experienced by the person on the other side of the table.

But death is natural, even when it isn't. It's a stage of life just like childhood, puberty, adolescence and adulthood. Having a conversation with your nearest and dearest, especially when times are calm, empowers not only you but everyone you care about to face the inevitable together one day.

A helping hand?

There are numerous places around the world where providing medical aid for terminally ill patients to die is legal. This is often called medically assisted death or assisted suicide. To my mind, assisted suicide seems an antiquated and odd turn of phrase, although it's commonly used: Google shows that people overwhelmingly search for assisted suicide rather than assisted dying.

The problem is the way we speak about something determines how we perceive it. An assisted death is a medical procedure in response to the harsh reality of various terminal illnesses. If we conflate assisted dying with suicide, it is at best misleading and at worst harmful.

Up until the late nineteenth century, suicide was criminalised in many places, particularly the US, where the deceased would have their property confiscated posthumously and would be denied a Christian burial. While suicide is no longer a criminal act in most countries, it still bears the burden of heavy stigma. When one hears or reads the word suicide it triggers dread, horror or shock and when we label assisted dying as suicide, we tap into those taboos and moral judgements.

This becomes harmful when terminally ill patients feel they have to hide their preference for an assisted death for fear of being judged by society

Death 2.0

or even close family. It can also make family members feel guilt and shame, and be understandably fearful of committing a crime in the eyes of the law.

A patient who is terminally ill and wants an assisted death doesn't necessarily want to die; if they had their terminal diagnosis reversed, they might not want to end their life. But if death is unavoidable, then it's a decision not between life and death but about the type of death you want: one where you are in control versus prolonged suffering without control.

On the surface, the argument for legalising assisted dying seems straightforward: people should have the right to choose how and when they die, particularly in cases of unbearable suffering with no chance of recovery. In a world where we champion autonomy in life, why should it suddenly vanish when facing death? But assisted dying is not just about individual choice, it's about the systems that surround that choice.

In an ideal world, assisted dying laws would only serve those who truly need them: people suffering from terminal, untreatable conditions who make a rational, well-informed decision to end their suffering. But we don't live in an ideal world. We live in a world where vulnerable people (disabled, elderly, people with severe mental health issues, or even the economically disadvantaged) could feel pressured into choosing death because they see themselves as a burden.

In addition, medical care is increasingly dictated by costs. In a struggling healthcare system, what happens when assisted dying becomes the cheaper, more convenient option? Once the door is opened, where does it stop? Countries like Canada and Belgium have seen criteria for assisted dying expand beyond terminal illness to mental health conditions and non-life-threatening disabilities.

The concern isn't just what happens if we allow this, it's how do we ensure it doesn't spiral into something unintended? For that reason, if assisted dying were to be legalised, it would need to be governed by rigorous regulation that centred on the rights and wishes of the patient.

This Is Vital Information

Who wants to live for ever?

On this Earth right now, approximately 100 billion people have lived and then died. Although some religions have put forward convincing proposals to the contrary, we don't have proof that any of these people have returned from an afterlife to confirm or deny its existence. To date, nobody has proven that cheating death is, in fact, possible. (If you're reading this in the year 4000 and have the technology to reverse death, please don't try to bring me back. I apologise for my cynicism.)

Until the sixteenth century, humankind considered death with a sense of resignation. Religion underpinned the sentiment that doctors shouldn't try to hold back death because it was the will of God. In the mid-1500s, the philosopher and statesman Sir Francis Bacon was among the first to suggest that medicine should combat death rather than passively accept it as divine will. It wasn't until the mid-1900s that we devised the means and medicine – like antibiotics and life-support technology – to delay the slow shuffle towards the edge of this mortal coil.

The modern fascination with preventing, cheating and reversing death has unsurprisingly facilitated the dawn of new (slightly dubious) industries, such as cryonics. The goal of cryopreservation is to preserve a human body by freezing it until a time that technology is available to bring that person back from the dead.

Proponents of cryonics equate the process to that of frozen embryos, which are reanimated after being frozen for decades. The difference is that a fully grown human adult and its accompanying brain is much larger and more complex than an embryo. The freezing process destroys and damages cells and tissues, not to mention neurons that facilitate memory or 'sense of self'. As of now, it is not viable to freeze someone and bring them back and even if we could, would it be worth it?

Others who want to prolong life include extropians, who subscribe to the philosophy of extropianism, which embraces human enhancement. They want to live longer and overcome limits like ageing or death with greater physical and mental health.

The problem with this utopian view is that DNA and every cell in our body comes with an expiry date. Mortality is hardwired and programmed into our very core. Balancing the immortality equation would require solving numerous biological problems. To break the age barrier of roughly 125 years, we would need to re-engineer our biology through artificial means.

There are also transhumanists who believe humans should enhance themselves using technology. Their aim is to transcend the evolutionary limitations of the human body, not merely by changing one's lifestyle but through external enhancements to our bodies. By incorporating technology, such as genetic engineering, into our flesh and bones, the goal is to control evolution and transform the human species into human 2.0.

Perhaps the simple answer is to transfer the information that encodes all our thought processes and memories from our brain on to a computer. As technology approaches the singularity (when artificial intelligence becomes so advanced it surpasses human intelligence), perhaps we can rid ourselves of tumours, genetic errors and decaying tissue by being at one with the machines? If we upload our consciousness into a server, perhaps we can live for ever until technology is at a point where we can 'body hop' and upgrade bodies like characters in a video game. Is that the true dystopian version of immortality?

Unfortunately, cells aren't built to last. With vaccines, agriculture, modern technology, diet, exercise and all other sorts of manipulations, we've already extended the warranty period well beyond its means. In short, evolution will always favour death. This shaky contract evolution has with the Grim Reaper means our bodies will become frailer beyond a certain timeframe. In fact, a study published in *Nature* in 2021 suggested that the human body is not capable of much more than 120 years of existence before cumulative DNA damage commits us to our doom.

This Is Vital Information

Seriously, who wants to live for ever?

As increasing numbers of people live to their eighties, nineties and even their one hundreds, we must ask ourselves: are we actually *extending* life, or simply prolonging death?

To answer this question, researchers from the Karolinska Institute made use of public databases to analyse the deaths of people in Sweden over the age of seventy between 2018 and 2020, aiming to find out *how* elderly people die – is it a long, drawn-out affair or a short sudden death? At home, fully compos mentis? Or physically and mentally impaired in their final days? Unfortunately, the finding suggested a disturbing weighting towards the latter.

This then begs the question, how can we have a 'better' death?

If I were to die tomorrow, I would want full control of my physical and mental senses and remain independent, be free of pain, have autonomy over where my final resting place would be and not have my life artificially prolonged to no good end.

Perhaps up until now in our quest to 'cure' ageing we have paid more attention to merely living longer (lifespan) rather than on the number of years in good physiological health, free of disability and chronic disease (health span). In an ideal world, we would achieve parity between both, but while we have extended our lifespan over the past few decades, the health span has not seen a similar rise. In fact, many studies done in the US, for example, suggest there is a gap of up to fifteen years between lifespan and health span: people live with suboptimal health for almost a decade and a half towards the end of their lives.

When it comes to end-of-life care, we are similarly fixated on increasing the lifespan with no concern for health span. While there are procedures that aid health in old age, like a cataract operation or a new hearing device, the best way to avoid poor health is to prevent debilitating conditions from rearing their heads in the first place. Unfortunately, much of this will sound familiar (but is also true): eat a balanced diet, don't smoke, avoid or moderate alcohol intake, have a good social network, challenge your brain, regulate stress and be physically active throughout life. Quite simply, the best chance of having a 'good' death is by living a good, healthy life.

A final thought

Well, here we are. You're officially dead. You had a good run, or maybe your turn was cut short – you batted your way through whatever innings you had and had a few highlights. You saw the Eiffel Tower, you got that car you always wanted, you saw Coldplay live, read all the Harry Potter books twice over . . . but you are dead. Don't beat yourself up, it happens to the best and worst of us.

As you lay there in the cadaverous environs of the hospital side room, or bitten in half by a great white shark, or sitting slumped on a toilet with your last act being a strenuous, high-strain dump, let me ask . . . was your last thought a good one?

To explore further how people perceive death I had an in-depth conversation with a palliative care nurse and asked her about the most common regrets she hears from people on their deathbeds. It probably comes as little shock that the one expressed, almost universally, was that they wished they hadn't worked so hard.

This is not to say that hard work and accumulating money is meaningless, as anyone who has struggled with finances will testify, but many studies have shown that the influence wealth has on happiness is not linear and has diminishing returns after our basic needs are met.

I'm not a philosopher nor a theologian but I do have frequent existential thoughts – that's normal, right? From the great thinkers of the past to this humble general surgeon, we're all in agreement that embracing death is a fundamental aspect of living life fully. The act of recognising the finitude of your life creates an angst that life is random, wonderful, a comedy show, awful, bizarre, peculiar, beautiful and both full of meaning and meaningless at the same time. We are brought into this world without a choice and we might disappear just as inexplicably as we arrived. In between, many of us feel obligated to conform to what the world expects of us rather than figuring what we want and how to make the most of life.

Another common deathbed regret people have is wishing they hadn't worried so much about the expectations and perceptions of others and lived a life truer to their own core beliefs and wants; that they had lived a more authentic life. Conforming to societal norms is easy because it is expected. It will 'feel' like the right thing to do and you'll be cajoled by those around you that you are indeed doing the right thing. In fact, turning from the path of conformity might incite resentment from friends and family, especially if you wander on to 'taboo' paths, as I found myself when I started balancing life both as a surgeon by day (and occasionally by night) as well as an online video creator. More than once I heard hushed discussions as I passed by. 'Surgeons shouldn't be making videos online . . .'

If I had listened to those voices, I might have carried on with my life in exactly the same way. That's OK – I was, after all, doing a pretty worthwhile job. But instead, I followed my instincts and the unconventional path I chose has brought me happiness and may have saved someone's life in the process. And that's all we can ask for, right?

Memento mori

Remember, you will die.

It might not be a phrase you'd immediately think of as fashionable, but this was the 'live, laugh, love' of the ancient world – scholars, military personnel, artists and everyday folk would have small souvenirs of skulls, hour-glasses or candles to illustrate mortality and to remind themselves of their eventual end.

You might even wonder why anyone would strive to be constantly reminded of death, if yearly tax returns weren't enough of a mood kill. It centres around a concept known as temporal scarcity. The rarer or scarcer

Death 2.0

a commodity is, whether it's a rare book or a cinnamon and pumpkin spiced mocha chai, the perceived value of this item rises. The same goes for life. The more we are reminded that time is in short supply, the more it is valued.

Outside the hospital I've tried to create my own 'death reminders' akin to memento mori. These make me aware of how much life I could have left, how grateful I should be for the time and experiences I've had, and to plan what else I can do.

One of the exercises I've done is count the number of summers I've had and the ones I potentially have left. You can count the number of weeks, the number of Tuesdays or whatever you find helps. If you tally it up, it might be that you have just forty more summers to go. Which means you have to figure out what you have to do or want to do before the end. It solidifies your plans and ambitions and pushes you to be more intentional in how you live your life, meaning you avoid being six feet under with a list of unfinished hopes and dreams.

So, let me ask you: what do you want to do with your summers?

ACKNOWLEDGEMENTS

To my wife and parents . . . the three pillars of patience holding up the temple of my questionable life choices. Also, for understanding that 'I'm just finishing one more paragraph' actually means 'See you next week'.

To Shadow, my dog, therapist, and co-author in spirit . . . who slept through every draft and still believed in me, mostly because I control his food supply. Shadow, thanks for reminding me that no matter how bad a day gets, someone will still enthusiastically sniff my shoes. He contributed nothing to the research but everything to my mental health and reminded me that sometimes all you need is unconditional love . . . and opposable thumbs.

And finally, to you . . . the people who watched, read, followed, commented, laughed, questioned, and cared. You've given me the rare gift of finding purpose beyond a scalpel. Together, we've built a space where curiosity trumps perfection and where education beats elitism . . . where health isn't measured in 5 a.m. yoga sessions, kale smoothies, or detox teas but in the courage to talk about the things we were told not to.

Thank you for listening. And for not unfollowing me when I mentioned poop for the hundredth time.

Thank you for letting me turn oversharing into a career and for proving that science, sarcasm, and sincerity can coexist.

Health and life is about understanding the messy, taboo, ridiculous human stuff we were never meant to talk about . . . until now.

TABLE OF **FODMAP** FOODS

	Low FODMAP	**High FODMAP**
Fruit	Banana, Blueberry, Cantaloupe, Cranberry, Grape, Kiwifruit, Lemon, Lime, Orange, Pineapple, Raspberry, Strawberry	Apple, Apricot, Avocado, Blackberry, Cherry, Date, Fig, Mango, Nectarine, Peach, Plum, Sultana, Tinned Fruit, Watermelon
Vegetables	Aubergine, Beansprouts, Carrot, Courgette, Cucumber, Lettuce, Olive, Pak Choy, Parsnip, Plantain, Radish, Spinach, Tomato, White Potato	Artichoke, Asparagus, Broccoli, Brussels Sprouts, Garlic, Leek, Mushroom, Okra, Onion, Sweet Potato, Sweetcorn
Breads, Cereals, Grains and Pasta	Cornflour, Crisps, Gluten-Free Breads and Pastas, Oats, Polenta, Pretzels, Quinoa, Rice	Barley, Bran, Cereal, Cous Cous, Granola, Muesli, Pasta, Rye, Semolina, Spelt, Wheat foods e.g. Bread
Milk Products (and alternatives)	Almond Milk, Butter, Cheddar, Cream, Crème Fraiche, Dark Chocolate, Edam, Feta, Goats Cheese, Lactose Free Milk, Mozzarella, Sorbet, Soya Custard, Soya Ice Cream	Buttermilk, Cows Milk, Goats Milk, Greek Yoghurt, Ice Cream, Processed Cheese, Ricotta, Sheeps Milk
Nuts and Seeds	Almonds, Coconut, Macadamia Nuts, Peanuts, Pecans, Sesame Seeds, Sunflower Seeds, Walnuts	Cashew, Pistachio
Other	Eggs, Maple Syrup, Peanut Butter, Tofu, Treacle	Agave, Honey, Protein Powders, Sugar-Free Chewing Gum

INDEX

Page references in *italics* indicate images.

Aché hunter-gatherers 57
acid mantle 55–6, 67
acid reflux 5, 48
acne 55, 56–9, 236
ACT (acceptance and commitment therapy) 279
ADHD (attention deficit hyperactivity disorder) 213, 230–33
adipokines 158
adrenaline 107, 217, 237, 238
adrenocorticotropic hormone (ACTH) 236
age 47, 88, 91, 105, 110
    anti-ageing products 57, 59, 60
    curing/longevity and 248, 286–9
    menopause and 78, 80, 82–3
    penis and 98–9
agoraphobia 14
alcohol 17, 25, 49, 51, 56, 84, 92, 103, 112, 146, 255, 256, 257, 262, 289
amputations 200–201, 208
anus 20, 73, 117, 118, 135, 142, 155
    anal sex 133–5, 142, 146, 151
    muscles/sphincter 2, 4, 18, 20, 21, 29, 73
    pain in 73
anxiety 95, 155, 167, 210
    ADHD and 231, 232, 233
    BDD and 201

BMI and 167
bowel opening and 3, 11, 14, 19
cognitive behavioural therapy (CBT) and 221
erection and 106, 107
hair loss and 119
IBS and 24, 25
menopause and 77
mental health and 213, 214, 215, 216–17, 218
personal failure, perception of/ healthcare professionals and 234, 235
physical manifestation of 235–6
physical health and 219, 220
stress and see stress
testosterone and 115
aphrodisiacs 105–106
appendectomy 233–4
archaea 19
atherosclerosis 98–9, 109, 115
axons 224–5

B cells 129
Bacon, Sir Francis 286
bacteria
    death and 276, 277
    gut and 7, 8, 10, 19, 20, 30, 31, 32, 33, 162, 276
    hygiene and 35–7, 41, 42, 48–9, 50, 102

Index

B cells – *cont.*
  oral 45, 46, 47
  skin and 52, 54–5, 57, 58
  vagina and 84
BDSM (bondage and discipline, dominance and submission, sadism and masochism) 154
beans 30, 31, 162
beta-carotene 174
beta-glucan 8, 10
Big Pharma 99, 263, 264
biotin 120, 121
bipolar disorder 213, 232
blue balls 136–8
BMI (body mass index) 167–9, 176, 182, 210
body modification *186*, 187–211
  amputations 200–201, 208
  bionic limbs controlled by brain signals 202
  body dysmorphic disorder (BDD) 201–202
  body integrity identity disorder (BIID) 200–202
  breast augmentation 207–208
  breast reduction/reduction mammoplasty 209–10
  cochlear implants 203
  foot binding 205–206
  heels 205, 206–207
  medical 202–204
  Otzi the Iceman 188–9, 192
  piercing *186*, 192–5, 199
  plastic surgery 207–11
  prosthetics 203, 204
  'restoration' and 'enhancement', blurred line between 203
  scars 195–9
  social media and 210–11
  tattoos 187, 188–92, 196, 199, 208
  weight and 211
body odour 35, 42–3
borborygmi (gut groans) 1–2
bowel 1–6, 8, 9, 11, 13, 15, 17–20, 70, 72, 73, 78, 79, 84, 117, 224
  cancer 4–5, 6, 46, 242, 249, 254, 260
  inflammatory bowel disease (IBD) 21, 24
  irritable bowel syndrome (IBS) 8, 23–7, 31
  parcopresis (shy bowel syndrome) 12, 14
brain
  ADHD and 230–31
  anxiety and 236
  beauty of 214
  BIID and 201
  bionic limbs controlled by signals in 202
  brain fog 79, 80
  cancer and 245, 260, 265
  death and 282, 286, 287, 289
  diet and 10, 161–2
  grief and 279–80
  gut-brain axis 16, 23, 25–7, 162, 163, 176
  hypothalamus 83, 113, 237
  inner workings of 224–9
  lobotomies 221–4
  menopause and 78, 79, 80, 83
  menstruation and 67–8
  mental health and 214, 215–16, 217, 220, 221–2
  mind and 226–9
  neural implants 203
  neurons 27, 133, 138, 153, 203, 221, 224–7, 229, 238, 239, 279, 286
  neurotransmitters 213, 219, 220, 221, 225–6, 231
  orgasm and 138, 139, 139–40
  pain and 90–91, 153–4
  penis and 104, 107–108, 139

Index

sleep and 239
stress and 113, 236, 237, 238
breasts 78
  augmentation 207–208
  cancer 81, 82, 87, 89–93, 190, 247, 252, 263, 266
  checking 89
  health 86–93
  normal 87–9
  pain 89–90
  reduction/reduction mammoplasty 209–10
breathing 27, 113, 130, 209, 237–8, 281, 282
Buisson, Odile 140
bulbospongiosus 117

calcium 85
cancer 241–68
  body MRI (magnetic resonance imaging) scan and 265–6
  bowel cancer 4–5, 6, 46, 242, 249, 254, 260
  breast cancer 81, 82, 87, 89–93, 190, 247, 252, 263, 266
  carcinogenic environmental factors 254–5
  cells, cancerous *240*
  cervical cancer 146, 147
  chemotherapy 46, 78, 249–51, 253, 254
  colorectal cancer 82, 123
  cure, why we can't 261
  defined 244–6
  endometrial cancer 82
  evolution of 249–50
  failing to overcome 262–7
  future of 259–61
  HPV and 146–7
  IARC classification for carcinogens 256–7
  immunotherapy and 252–3
  longevity and 248
  lung cancer 87
  news of 241–2
  oral cancer 49, 50, 146–8
  oropharyngeal cancer 146–8
  pancreatic cancer 241, 242
  prevention 261–2
  radiotherapy 78, 250–54
  screening 5, 259, 260, 261, 262, 263, 264, 266, 267
  scrotal cancer in chimney sweeps 255
  skin cancer 60, 242, 255
  smoking and 49, 50
  talking about 246–8
  targeted therapy 252
  tell-tale signs of 249
  testicular cancer 258–9
  throat cancer 145, 146–8
  treating 249, 250–54
  word 242–3
carbohydrates 8, 31, 48, 161, 175, 176
cardiovascular health 46, 47, 80, 81, 86, 106, 109, 159, 160, 165, 170, 176, 184, 247, 265
cellulite 180–82
Centers for Disease Control and Prevention (CDC), US 146
central nervous system *212*
ceramides 55, 85
cervical cancer 146, 147
chemotherapy 46, 78, 249–51, 253, 254
childbirth 37–8
cholecystokinin 9, 163
cholesterol 7, 8, 86, 108, 115, 169, 170
'clinically proven' 59
clitoris 63, 64, *122*, 139, 140
cochlear implants 203, 204
coeliac disease 31, 179

Index

coffee 9, 16, 43, 47, 51, 72, 118, 153, 177, 181, 256, 273
cognitive behavioural therapy (CBT) 83, 220, 221, 279
colonic adaptation 30
constipation 4, 15–17, 21–2, 23, 26, 28, 72, 73, 84, 117, 176
contraception 71, 82, 126
corpora cavernosa 104, 135, 136
corticotropin-releasing hormone (CRH) 236
cortisol 106, 107, 112–13, 119, 129, 164, 227, 236, 237, 238
Covid-19 37, 152
cramps 65, 70–71, 73, 74, 76
Cronin, Thomas 208
cryonics 286
CT scan 6, 13, 45, 76, 131, 170, 234, 241
curry 11
cyclic guanosine monophosphate (cGMP) 106
cysteine 32
Czerny, Vincenz 208

dairy products 8, 14, 31, 32, 111
death 269–91
  'better' 288
  body after 273–4
  cafés 273
  dying wishes 281–4
  grief 269–72, 277–80
  health span 288–9
  longevity and 286–9
  medicalisation of 280–81
  medically assisted death or assisted suicide 284–5
  microbiome 276–7
  mortality salience (dwelling on the subject) 273

preventing, cheating and reversing, modern fascination with 285–6
primary flaccidity 274
reminders 291
regrets, common 289–90
rigor mortis 274–6
SPIKES protocol 270–71
talking about 272–3
dentistry 43–6, 50–51
depression 25, 27, 48, 115, 167, 210, 213, 215, 219–22, 227–31, 233, 278
dermatology 55, 57–60, 198
desquamation 54–5
diarrhoea 1–3, 19, 23, 28, 71, 73, 216, 251
diet 48–9, 171–9
  acne and 57
  best 171–2, 177
  cancer and 251, 255, 262, 267
  complex 179
  death and 287, 289
  'detox' 178
  fad 173
  fat and see fat
  fibre and see fibre
  FODMAP 8, 25, 295
  gut/faeces and 7, 9, 16, 17, 19, 21, 22, 25, 66, 84–5
  hair loss and 120
  keto 175
  menopause and 81, 84–5, 86
  paleo 175
  penis and 105
  plant-based 9–11, 85, 169, 173, 175–8
  raw food 173–4
  scars and 199
  severe dietary restrictions as enemy of long-term goals 178
  simplicity of 177

Index

sleep diet 164
vegan 172, 176, 176–7
weight loss and see weight loss
digestive tract 16, 33, 46
dihydrostestosterone (DHT) 119, 120, 121
DNA 53, 146, 187, 229, 244, 245, 251, 254, 255, 257, 287
dopamine 154, 213, 226, 231, 238
Douglas, Charlene 139–41
Douglas, Michael 145–6, 147, 148
dysbiosis 49–50, 84

Egyptians, ancient 192
endometriosis 75–7, 155
endorphins 71, 129, 130, 153, 238
endothelium 109
erection 96, 101, 104–18, 135–7, 138
   brain and 107–109
   detumescence 117
   diet and 105
   erectile dysfunction (ED) 99, 104–109, 114, 117, 120, 123, 136
   morning glory 106–107
   pelvic floor muscles and 117–18
   sleep and 106
   testosterone and 110–11
   weight and 109–10
evolution 90, 91, 100, 102, 125–7, 131, 237, 250, 258, 259, 287
exfoliation 54, 58, 60, 121
extropians 286–7

faeces 1–33, 41, 53, 132
   bowel motions 11–18
   constipation 4, 15–17, 21–3, 26, 28, 72, 73, 84, 117, 176
   diarrhoea 1–3, 19, 23, 28, 71, 73, 216, 251
   diet and 7–11
   facts 6–7
   faecal impaction 13
   holidays and 19–20
   periods and 71–3
   poo cushion 12
   poo normal 17–18
   poo problems 20–28
   poo routine 15
   rectum and 18–19
   See also gut
farting/flatulence 6, 21, 28–33
fat 157–85
   body fat percentage 168, 171
   BMI (body mass index) 167–9, 176, 182, 210
   cellulite 180–81
   diets and 160–61, 171–9
   exercise and 160
   GLP–1 and 162–3
   healthy 10, 65, 85, 86, 120, 164
   layers in the stomach *156*
   money from, history of making 166
   obesity and see obesity
   penis and 109
   reducing 160–61
   society and 182–4
   sleep and 164
   Sumo wrestlers 169–70
   trans 184
   visceral 109, 159–61, 164, 165, 168, 169–70
   waist-to-hip ratio (WHR) 168
   weight and 92, 157–61 see also weight/weight-loss
   women, body fat in 171
female health. *See* women
fibre 7–10, 17, 20, 21, 22, 23, 30, 31, 43, 48–9, 66, 85, 161–3, 173, 174, 176, 276

Index

fight-or-flight response 130, 237
finasteride 120, 121
5-alpha reductase 119, 120
flavanols 9, 10
Flush Hush 11–12
fMRI scan 138, 239
FODMAPs (fermentable oligo-, di-, mono-saccharides and polyols) 8, 25, *295*
food diary 14, 25
food intolerances 18
foot binding 187, 205–206
foot stools 17
Fordyce spots 100
Freeman, Walter 222–4
Fructooligosaccharides (FOS) 8
FUE (follicular unit extraction) 120
fusobacterium 46
FUT (follicular unit transplantation) 120

G-spot 138, 140–41
Galactooligosaccharides (GOS) 8
Gardasil 147
gastrocolic effect 9
gastrointestinal (GI) tract 46
genetics 47, 56, 91, 119, 125–6, 160, 168, 171, 182, 214, 245, 253, 255, 261, 287. See also DNA
genitalia, female external 62, 64, 65
Gerow, Frank 208
ginseng 99
glial cells 224
GLP-1 161–3, 165
gluten 179
gonorrhoea 130, 141–2, 143, 152
Google 27–8, 174, 182, 266, 284
Gräfenberg, Ernst 140
Greeks, ancient 22–3, 64, 96, 115, 126, 189, 192, 217–18

grief
  five stages of 277–9
  neuroscience of 279–80
  SPIKES protocol and 270–71
guanylate cyclase 106
gut
  constipation and see constipation
  faeces and 1–28 see *also* faeces
  flatulence and 28–33
  gut-brain axis 16, 23, 25–7, 162, 163, 176
  menopause and 84–5
  microbiome 7, 9, 10, 19, 20, 49, 84, 219, 256, 276
  prebiotics and see prebiotics
  probiotics and see probiotics

haemorrhoids *viii*, 4, 20–23, 73, 127, 133–4
hair loss 118–21, 251
Haji, Amou (world's dirtiest man) 39–40
handwashing 37–9, 40
health span 288–9
heels 205, 206–207
herpes 143, 144–5
Hippocrates 22–3, 218
HIV 148–52
  nail salons and 150
  PEP (post-exposure prophylaxis) 150–52
  PrEP (pre-exposure prophylaxis) 151–2
  transmission of 148–9
  what to do if you think you have been exposed to 149
holidays, gut and 19–20
hormones
  acne and 56–7
  breasts and 88–9, 91, 92
  fat and 158, 159, 161, 162, 163–4, 165, 170

Index

hormonal contraception 71
   IBS and 23
   menopause and 78, 79, 80–82, 83
   mental health and 236
   penis and 106, 107, 109–15
   sex and 130
   stress and 107, 113, 129, 227, 236
horny goat weed 99–100
HPA (hypothalamic-pituitary-adrenal) axis 237
HPV (human papillomavirus) 145–8, 245
'humours', four 218
Hunter, John 141–2
hyaluronic acid 85
hydrogen sulphide 32, 277
hygiene 16, 33, 35–61, 67, 73, 119, 150, 203, 204
   body odour 42–3
   handwashing 37–9
   immune system and 36–7, 39, 40, 47, 54, 58
   mouth/oral health 43–51 see also mouth
   pubic hair and 100–102
      shoes inside the house 35–6
   showering 40–42
   skin 34, 52–61
   sleep 83
   teeth 43–51 see also teeth
   world's dirtiest man (Amou Haji) 39
hypnotherapy 26–7
'hypoallergenic' 59
hypothalamus 83, 113, 237

immune system 174, 188, 191, 194, 197
   cancer and 245, 250, 252–3
   fibre and 7, 30
   gut 26
   HIV and 151
   HPV and 146
   hygiene and 36, 39, 40, 47, 54
   immunoglobulin A (IgA) 129
   immunotherapy 252–3, 254
   microbiome and 276
   sex and 128–30
   stress and 58, 145, 219
imperfection 233–6
inflammation 5, 10, 21, 22, 47, 49, 68, 71, 72, 196, 216, 234, 236
   cancer and 245
   depression and 229–30
   diet and 174, 179
   exercise and 57–8
   fat and 158, 169
   menopause and 84–6
   penis and 109, 110
   sex and 129, 155
   weight and 92
inflammatory bowel disease (IBD) 21, 24
inhaler 50
International Agency for Research on Cancer (IARC) classification for carcinogens 256–7
iproniazid 229
iron 16, 28, 69, 119, 176–7, 232
irritable bowel syndrome (IBS) 8, 23–7, 31
ischiocavernosus 104, 117
IVF (in vitro fertilisation) 126–7

Jannini, Emmanuele 140
Japan 12, 96, 189

Karna Vedha 192
Karolinska Institute 288
Kegel exercises 118
Kennedy, Rosemary 222–3
keto diet 175

Index

Kinsey, Alfred: *Sexual Behavior in the Human Male* 127–8
Kitavan tribes, Papua New Guinea 57
kiwi fruit 17
Kolletschka, Jakob 38
Komisaruk, Barry 138–9
Kübler-Ross, Elisabeth 278

La Bicêtre asylum, Paris 218
laxatives 17, 165
libido 64, 106, 109, 110, 114, 120, 126
lifespan 172, 254, 288–9
lignans 9, 10
Lindsay, Timmie Jean 208
lobotomies 221–4
longevity 248, 286–9
love 30
lycopene (tomatoes) 174
Lyman, Monty 52

macrophages 129, 188, 191
male health 95–121
   hair loss *see* hair loss
   penis *see* penis
   pelvic floor muscles *see* pelvic floor muscles
   prostate *see* prostate
   reproductive system, male *122*
   testosterone *see* testosterone
mansplaining 65, 79–80, 93
marijuana 111–12
medicalisation of death 280–81
medically assisted death or assisted suicide 284–5
medication 16, 27, 32, 47–8, 57, 74, 78, 99, 105, 108, 114, 120, 151, 163, 165, 219–21, 227, 250, 251
menopause 77–86, 91, 155, 178
   brain fog and 80

   disease classification and 80
   gut health/diet and 84–5
   hormones and 80–82
   HRT (hormone replacement therapy) 81
   medical definition of 78
   menopause hormone therapy (MHT) 81–3
   one-year anniversary 79
   ovulation ending and 79
   perimenopause 63, 64, 78, 79, 80, 81, 178
   physical activity and 86
   post-menopause 85, 178
   reverse puberty rollercoaster 79
   skincare and 85–6
   sleep and 83–4
   Women's Health Initiative (WHI) and 82–3
mental health 27, 119, 155, 165, 196, 199, 201, 210, 213–40, 285, 287
   ADHD (attention deficit hyperactivity disorder) 213, 230–33
   adrenocorticotropic hormone (ACTH) 236
   anxiety *see* anxiety
   attitudes to 219–21
   awareness of 215–16
   bipolar disorder 213, 232
   borderline personality disorder 213
   brain and 214, 215–16, 217, 220, 221–2
   breath and 237–8
   central nervous system *212*
   cognitive behavioural therapy (CBT) 83, 220, 221, 279
   corticotropin-releasing hormone (CRH) and 236
   defined 215–17
   depression *see* depression
   history of 217–19

Index

'If you hear hoof beats, think horses, not zebras' 216–17
imperfection and 233–6
institutions for the mentally ill 218
lobotomies 220–24
medication 219–21, 227, 228, 229
obsessive-compulsive disorder (OCD) and 213, 222
physical health and 219
psychotherapy 27, 83, 120, 202, 219–21
schizophrenia and 213, 222
serotonin and 213, 220, 221, 226, 228–30, 238
sleep and 239
SSRIs (selective serotonin reuptake inhibitors) 220, 221, 228, 229
stigma 213, 218, 220, 221, 230, 232
stress and see stress
supernatural explanations for 218
microbiome 173, 256
  death and 276–7
  gut 9, 10, 19, 20, 49, 84, 219, 256
  immune system and 36, 40
  oral 49, 51
  skin 55, 56, 57, 58
  vagina 66, 67
minoxidil 119, 120, 121
moisturisers 59, 60, 198
Monash University, Australia 31
Moniz, Egas 222
morning glory 106–107
mortality salience 273
Mortensen, Helen 223–4
mouth/oral health 43–51
  HPV and 146–7
  mouthwash 43, 46, 51
  oral bugs 46–7
  pH level 48–50
  teeth 43–51 see also teeth

xerostomia (dry mouth) 48
MRI (magnetic resonance imaging) scan 77, 98, 138, 154, 210, 230, 239, 265–7

narrowed arteries 107
natty [natural] or not debates 115
natural killer (NK) cells 129
natural moisturising factors (NMFs) 54
neural implants 203
neurons 27, 133, 138, 153, 203, 221, 224–7, 229, 238, 239, 279, 286
neuroscience. See brain
neurotransmitters 213, 219, 220, 221, 225–6, 231
nitric oxide 99, 100, 105, 106, 108, 109
'non-comedogenic' 59
NSAID (non-steroidal anti-inflammatory drug) 71, 74
nucleus accumbens 154
nutrition labels 184

obesity 57, 109, 158, 159, 166–7, 170, 182, 185
obsessive-compulsive disorder (OCD) 213, 222
odour 18–19, 30, 31–2, 35, 42–3, 67
oligosaccharide 8, 31
omega-3 fatty acids 10, 65, 86, 120
oral sex 142, 144–7
orgasm 117, 123, 129, 130, 136–7, 138–40
oropharyngeal cancers 146–7
Osler, William 23
Otzi the Iceman 188–9, 192
oxytocin 129, 130, 226

pain 47
  backside 73–4
  body modification and 205–10
  brain and 90–91, 153–4

Index

pain – *cont.*
   breast and 89–92
   endometriosis 73–6
   periods and 69–71
   pleasure and 153–5
   sex 77, 79, 153–5
paleo diet 172, 173, 174–5, 211
pancreatic cancer 241–2
Papua New Guinea 57, 196
parcopresis (shy bowel syndrome) 12, 14
paruresis (shy bladder syndrome) 14
pelvic floor muscles 16, 17, 21, 73, 74, 117–18, 155
penis 94, 95–118
   age and 98–9
   aphrodisiacs and 105–106
   brain and 107–108
   broken 135–6
   bulbospongiosus and 117
   curves, bends and banana shapes 101
   erection 96, 101, 104–18, 120, 123, 135–7, 138 see *also* erection
   Fordyce spots 100
   history of 96
   ischiocavernosus and 117
   male reproductive system 94
   names for 95
   pearly penile papules (PPP) 100
   pelvic floor muscles and 117–18
   phallic adoration 96
   prostate and 116
   pubic hair 101–103
   size 96–8
   sleep and 106
   supplements and 99–100
   suspensory ligament 98
   testosterone and 110–15
   testicles see testicles
   torn frenulum 124–5
   veins 101
PEP (post-exposure prophylaxis) 150–52
perimenopause 63–4, 78, 79, 80, 81
periodontitis 47, 49
periods, or menstruation 64, 67–75, 76, 77, 78, 79, 171, 253
Peyronie's disease 98
Phosphodiesterase-5 (PDE5) 106
physical activity 57–8, 71, 80, 85, 86, 92, 113, 138, 159–60, 170, 171, 181, 238, 255, 267, 287
physiotherapy 27, 209, 210
piercing *186*, 192–5, 199, 204
plant-based diets 9–11, 85, 169, 173, 175–8
plastic surgery 207–11
polyphenols 9, 10, 84, 174
Pott, Percivall 255
prebiotics 7–8, 56
PrEP (pre-exposure prophylaxis) 148, 151–2
primary flaccidity 274
Prince Albert (piercing) 193
probiotics 10, 20, 56, 84
proctalgia fugax 73–4
prostate 116, 117, 140, 155, 247, 248
prosthetics 203, 204
protein 7, 17, 31, 32, 85, 119, 120, 163, 178, 199, 251
psychotherapy 27, 120, 202, 219–21
pubic hair 101–103

radiotherapy 78, 250, 251–4
raffinose 31
rainbow, eating the 9–11, 179
raw food diet 173–4
rectum 4, 13, 14, 17–22, 28, 29, 73, 82, 123, 116, 131–5, 249
REM (rapid eye movement) 107, 265

Index

reproduction/reproductive system 76, *94*, 126–8, 131
resistant starch 8, 10, 32
retinoids 57, 85, 198
rigor mortis 274–6
Rodman, Dennis 135
Roland le Sarcere (Roland the Farter) 29
Romans, ancient 96, 189, 192
Rome criteria 24
Rome Foundation 5, 24
rosemary oil 121
Rutgers University 138

Salem witch trials, New England (1692) 218
salmonella 19
scars 166, 195–9
schizophrenia 213, 222
School of Public Health, Tehran 39
science-washing 58–9
scrotal cancer 255
sebum 42, 53–5, 65, 194, 236
seeds 11
Semmelweis, Ignaz 37–8
serotonin 27, 213, 220, 221, 226, 228–9, 238
sex 77, 79, 97, 99–100, 105, 123–56, 192–3, 208, 228, 247, 253, 258
    anal sex 133–5, 142, 146, 151
    BDSM 154
    blue balls 136–8
    clitoris *122*, 139, 140
    contraception 71, 82, 123
    culture and 126
        evolution of 125–6
    female ejaculation 140–41
    G-spot 138, 140–41
    haemorrhoids 127, 133–4
    herpes 143, 144–5
    HIV 148–52

HPV 145–8
immune system and 128–30
IVF (in vitro fertilisation) 126
Kinsey and 127–8
orgasm 117, 123, 129, 130, 136–7, 138–40
pain and pleasure 153–5
painful 77, 79, 154–5
penis and see penis
reproduction and 126
sacred and forbidden 126
sexually transmitted infection (STIs) 100, 123, 130, 131, 141–3, 148, 150, 152, 155
sleep and 130–31
shoes inside the house 35–6
showering 40–43
silicone
    gel 198
    injections 208
simethicone 32
sitz bath 22
Sjögren's syndrome 48
skin *34*, 52–61
    acid mantle 55–6, 67
    acne 55, 56–9, 236
    anatomy 62
    desquamation 54–5
    hygiene 53
    -lightening products 60–61
    menopause and 85–6
    microbiome 40–41, 55, 56, 57, 58
    natural moisturising factors (NMFs) 54
    retinoid and 57
    routine 53–4
    scars and 196–9
    science-washing and 58–9
    sebum 54–5
    shower and 41–2

Index

skin – *cont.*
- skincare rules 59–60
- tattoos and 188
- vagina and 65–6, 67

sleep
- cognitive behavioural therapy for insomnia (CBT–I) 83
- diet and 164, 171
- erection and 106–107
- hair loss and 121
- hygiene 83
- melatonin and 83
- menopause 79, 80, 83–4
- mental health and 219, 227, 232, 239
- REM, or rapid eye movement 107, 265
- schedule 83
- sex and 130–31, 145
- stress and 113, 239
- testosterone and 119

Smith, Robert 202
smoking 44, 47, 49, 50, 92, 108–109, 119, 146, 200, 245, 255, 257, 260, 262, 289
smoothie 10, 22, 91, 185
snake oil 121, 181
social media 22, 25, 39, 40, 61, 64, 81, 111, 115, 135, 149, 158, 163, 172, 210–11, 215, 231, 232
Solomon, Sheldon 273
sorbitol 16, 17
soup 11, 177, 243
spices 11, 84
SPIKES protocol 270–71
SSRIs (selective serotonin reuptake inhibitors) 220, 221, 228, 229
St Mary Bethlehem ('Bedlam') 219
steroids 7, 58, 114, 115, 198
stigma 12, 63–5, 70, 124, 134, 146–8, 155, 158, 167, 189, 203, 213, 218, 220–21, 230, 232, 284

Strachan, David 36
streptococcus 37, 46, 48
stress 16, 86, 112–13, 236–9, 289
- acne and 57–8
- breathing and 237–8
- cortisol and 106, 107, 112–13, 119, 129, 164, 227, 236, 237, 238
- hair loss and 120
- herpes and 145
- IBS and 24–5
- mental health and 214, 216, 217, 218, 219, 227, 229, 236–9
- penis and 106, 107
- physical activity 238
- physiology of 237
- sleep and 239
- weight and 164, 169, 171

stroke 5, 115, 247
Sue, Jean-Joseph 200–201
sumo wrestlers 169–70
sunlight 58, 111
sunscreen 60, 198, 257
supplements 22, 31, 67, 81, 83, 99–100, 121, 176
supratentorial condition 24–5
sympathetic nervous system 130, 237
syphilis 142, 143, 152–3

tattoos 187, 188–91, 196, 208
tax 183, 184, 236, 246, 290
teeth 43–51, 199, 210
TENS (transcutaneous electrical nerve stimulation) machine 71
testicles
- blue balls 136–8
- prostate and 116
- testicular cancer 258–9
- testosterone and 110, 111, 115
- uneven 101

Index

testosterone 98–9, 108–15, 119
  abuse 115
  dihydrostestosterone (DHT) 119, 120, 121
  hair loss and 119
  low levels of 110–13
  treatments 113–15
throat cancer 145, 147
toilets 1, 2, 3, 4, 11, 12, 13, 14–17, 21–3, 26, 60, 144, 253, 289
tomatoes 9, 11, 174, 243
TOTO Sound Princess 12
transhumanism 287
Trump, Donald 152
tuberculosis 229–30, 248
tunica albuginea 104, 135–6

vagina 63, 65–8, 79, 139–40, 142, 155
vagus nerve 26, 27, 129, 139, 237
vaping 49–50
Vaseline 60
vegan diet 172, 175, 176–7
vegetables 9, 11, 20, 32, 49, 66, 105, 108, 162, 174, 184, 255, 256, 257
Viagra 99, 105, 106, 118
vitamins 7
  A 174
  B7 121
  B12 176
  C 177, 199
  cooking and 173
  D 58, 85, 111
vulva 63–7, 140

weight/weight loss 24, 43, 77, 92, 98, 157–86, 206, 207, 209, 211, 241, 249
  appetite regulation 161, 162, 163–4
  BMI (body mass index) and 167–9, 176, 182, 210
  cellulite and 180–81
  diets and 171–9 see also diets
  erection and 109–10
  fat and see fat
  fibre and 161–3, 173, 174, 176
  GLP-1 161–3, 165
  gluten and 179
  gut and 161, 163, 173, 176
  nutrition labels 184
  obesity see obesity
  society and 182–4
  weight-loss drugs 161–5
Whipple, Dr Beverly 139
Wilkes University, Pennsylvania 129, 130
women
  body modification see body modification
  breasts see breasts
  cellulite 180–81
  foot binding 187, 205–206
  genitalia, external 62, 64, 65
  health 63–93
  menopause see menopause
  periods, or menstruation see periods, or menstruation
  sex and see sex
  vagina see vagina
  weight-loss 165, 168, 171
Woodward, Dr Theodore 216
World Health Organization (WHO) 144, 184

xerostomia (dry mouth) 48

Yale Bereavement Study 278